Nishant Kumar

Perspectives on the Dynamic Behavior of Oral Lichen Planus

Nishant Kumar

Perspectives on the Dynamic Behavior of Oral Lichen Planus

What Dental Practitioners need to know

LAP LAMBERT Academic Publishing

Imprint

Any brand names and product names mentioned in this book are subject to trademark, brand or patent protection and are trademarks or registered trademarks of their respective holders. The use of brand names, product names, common names, trade names, product descriptions etc. even without a particular marking in this work is in no way to be construed to mean that such names may be regarded as unrestricted in respect of trademark and brand protection legislation and could thus be used by anyone.

Cover image: www.ingimage.com

Publisher:
LAP LAMBERT Academic Publishing
is a trademark of
International Book Market Service Ltd., member of OmniScriptum Publishing Group
17 Meldrum Street, Beau Bassin 71504, Mauritius

ISBN: 978-3-659-48489-6

Zugl. / Approved by: Meerut, Swami Vivekanand Subharti University, Library Dess., 2012

Copyright © Nishant Kumar
Copyright © 2013 International Book Market Service Ltd., member of OmniScriptum Publishing Group

ACKNOWLEDGEMENT

*I express my thanks and appreciation to my parents Dr. **Arun Kumar** and **Mrs. Gunjana Arun** and my brother **Sushant Kumar** for their understanding, motivation, efforts and unending love without which this job would have been impossible.*

*I would like to express my deepest appreciation to my guide **Dr. V. Sreenivasan**, who has the attitude and substance of a genius: I will always be indebted to him for his immense support.*

*It gives me great pleasure in acknowledging the support and help of **Dr. Prashant Patil**,. I express my sincere appreciation to him for his guidance and insight.*

*In addition a special thanks to **Dr. Sumit Goel**, who introduced me to linguistics and whose enthusiasm for the underlying structure, had lasting effect.*

*I express my deep gratitude and obligation to **Dr. Nikhil Srivastava**. Thanks go to **Dr. Shirin Vashishth** and **Dr. Swati Goel** for their valuable suggestions and comments especially when I needed it most.*

*Lastly, but in no sense the least, I am thankful to all colleagues and friends, **Dr. Ankit Goel** and **Dr. Sameer Rastogi** who made my work a memorable and valuable experience.*

CONTENTS

Sl.	Particular	Page No.
1.	Introduction	1 – 3
2.	General Concept	4 – 5
3.	Hypothesized Mechanisms	6 – 23
4.	Other Possible Mechanisms Of Pathogenesis of OLP	24 – 30
5.	Unifying Hypothesis to the Pathogenesis of OLP	31 – 40
6.	New Prospective to the Understanding of OLP	41 – 45
7.	Is OLP is a Pre-Malignant disease	46 – 48
8.	Detailed Aspect of Treatment	49
9.	Therapeutic approach based on the new concept	50
10.	Conclusion	51
11.	Figures	52 - 59
12.	Abbreviation	60
13.	References	61 - 72

INTRODUCTION

Lichen planus (LP) is a chronic inflammatory mucocutaneous disorder. *Lichen* comes from the Greek word leichen, meaning flat, and possibly the striking clinical colour of the pimples on skin led to the designation leichen ruber (latin; red). *Planus* refers to the clinical appearance of the skin papule; flattened, smooth and depressed on the summit, as first described by Wilson in 1869[1]. Although first described almost 150 years ago, and more than 5200 papers were present in the database Pub Med in January 2010, many aspects of the pathogenesis of LP are yet not fully understood.

The oral form of lichen planus (OLP) seems more common, chronic, and recalcitrant than the cutaneous type. The estimated prevalence of the disease in the general population is vary from 0.5% to 2.2%[2]. Fifty percent of patients with skin lesions also manifest oral mucosal lesions, and 25% of patients with OLP present only oral lesions. The disease has its peak incidence in the 30-60 years age range and has a female predominance of 2:1. OLP causes bilateral white striations, papules, or plaques on the buccal mucosa, tongue, and gingiva[3].

A wide clinical manifestation of OLP includes Reticular type, in which fine whitish striae crosses the mucosa; atrophic type, in which erythematous areas are surrounded by reticular components; Erosive type, exhibiting erythematous regions; Plaque type, and rarely bullous type. The OLP may present periods of remission, when the signs and symptoms are reduced or disappear and period of exacerbation, which may only be related to emotional distress.[4]

Since Erasmus Wilson describing of the disease in 1869, there has been a long controversy over the pathogenesis of the disease. Role of micro-organism in OLP has been studied by several authors. Chainani–Wu N et al concluded that there is association between OLP and HCV particularly in Spanish, Italian and Japanese population but no association is seen in British and Chinese population[5]. Yildirim B et al with their study concluded that there might be association of Epstein Barr virus (EBV) and Human Papilloma virus (HPV) with OLP however Herpes Simplex virus (HSV) does not seems to be associated[6]. Burkhart NW et al with their study suggested that there might be relationship between stress and oral lichen planus[7]. Carrozzo M et al concluded that HLA-DR6 may be responsible for the peculiar geographic heterogeneity of association between HCV and OLP thereby suggesting a genetic role in the disease[8]. However, according to Porter SR et al, OLP does not have a strong immunogenetic basis[9]. Yarom N et al believed that OLP carries an increased risk for chromosomal instability so has been supported by others[10].

Current data suggest that oral lichen planus is a T-cell–mediated autoimmune disease in which auto cytotoxic CD8+ T cells trigger apoptosis of oral epithelial cells. The dense sub-epithelial mononuclear infiltrate in oral lichen planus is composed of T cells and macrophages, and there are increased numbers of intra-epithelial T cells. Most T cells in the epithelium and adjacent to the damaged basal keratinocytes are activated CD8+ lymphocytes. Therefore, early in the formation of oral lichen planus lesions, CD8+ T cells may recognize an antigen associated with the major histocompatibility complex (MHC) class I on keratinocytes. After antigen recognition and activation, CD8+ cytotoxic T cells may trigger keratinocyte apoptosis. Activated CD8+ T cells (and possibly keratinocytes) may release cytokines that attract additional lymphocytes into the developing lesion[11].

OLP is unlikely to be caused by a single antigen but likely to be common outcome of the influence of a limited combination of extrinsic antigens, altered self antigens or super antigens. Various precipitating factors identified and enumerated by authors are dental restorative materials (amalgam, composites, resin, cobalt and gold), drugs (NSAIDs, ACE inhibitors), stress and infectious agents (HCV, HPV, CMV and EBV) [12]. We consider cause of OLP to be a complex and multifactorial which is associated with cytokine expression. Altogether, this makes the etiology behind OLP a multifactorial process comprising events that may take place at different time points.

Few questions have generated more controversy and passionate debate over the pathogenesis of the disease:-

1. Why and how does T cell accumulate in the superficial lamina propria in OLP?
2. Why and how T cell does enters in the oral epithelium in OLP?
3. What triggers keratinocyte apoptosis in OLP?
4. What is the role of micro-organism in OLP?
5. What is the role of stress in OLP?
6. Role of Genetics in OLP?

This Library Dissertation is an effort to clearly understand the pathogenesis of OLP and propose a unifying hypothesis for the pathogenesis of OLP.

GENERAL CONCEPT

Many controversies exist about the pathogenesis of oral lichen planus (OLP). Despite recent advances in understanding the immunopathogenesis of oral lichen planus (LP), the initial triggers of lesion formation and the essential pathogenic pathways are unknown. Evidences support a role of immune dysregulation in the pathogenesis. Certain things are clear from the histological features of OLP about the pathogenesis which is increased number of intra-epithelial lymphocytes, and degeneration of basal keratinocytes. Degenerating basal keratinocytes form colloid bodies that appear as homogenous eosinophilic globules. The ultra structure of colloid bodies suggests that they are apoptotic keratinocytes. The basal keratinocyte anchoring elements (hemidesmosomes, filaments, and fibrils) are disrupted in OLP. Degeneration of basal keratinocytes and disruption of the epithelial basement membrane and basal keratinocyte anchoring elements in OLP produce weaknesses at the epithelial connective tissue interface which may result in histological cleft formation and, rarely, clinical blistering of the oral mucosa (bullous lichen planus). Parakeratosis, acanthosis, and "saw-tooth" rete peg formation may be seen. B-cells and plasma cells are infrequent in OLP, and immunoglobulin and complement deposits are not a consistent feature [13] (Figure 1).

The inflammatory infiltrate consists primarily of T cells and macrophages. Plasma cells are rarely seen and immune deposits are not characteristic. In oral OLP, the majority of T cells within the epithelium and adjacent to damaged basal keratinocytes are activated CD8+ lymphocytes, while CD8+ T cells co-localize with apoptotic keratinocytes in oral LP lesions. T-cell lines and clones isolated from lichen planus lesions are more cytotoxic against autologous lesional keratinocytes than T-cell lines and clones from clinically normal skin of LP patients[11]. The majority of cytotoxic clones from LP lesions are CD8+ and the majority of non-cytotoxic clones are CD4+ (Figure 2). The cytotoxic activity of CD8+ lesional T-cell clones is partially inhibited by anti-MHC class I monoclonal antibody. These data suggest that CD8+ lesional T cells may be activated, at least in part, by an antigen associated with MHC class I on basal keratinocytes and that activated CD8+cytotoxic T cells may trigger keratinocyte apoptosis in oral LP. The nature of the antigen is uncertain. While the majority of intraepithelial lymphocytes in oral LP are CD8+, most lymphocytes in the lamina propria are CD4+. T-cell clones with helper activity and CD4+ T-cell clones that lack cytotoxic activity can be isolated from oral and cutaneous LP lesions, respectively. There are increased numbers of Langerhans cells (LCs) in oral LP lesions with up-regulated MHC class II expression. Keratinocytes in oral LP also express MHC class II antigens.[14]

HYPOTHESIZED MECHANISMS

The various mechanisms hypothesized to be involved in immune-pathogenesis are:-

A. Antigen-specific cell-mediated immune response

B. Non-specific mechanisms

C. Autoimmune response

D. Humoral immunity

Antigen Specific Cell Mediated Immune Response:-

The lymphocytic infiltrate in OLP is composed almost exclusively of T-cells and the majority of T-cells within the epithelium and adjacent to damaged basal keratinocytes are activated CD8+ lymphocytes. Analysis of data suggests that CD8+ T-cells are involved in disease pathogenesis, and that activated CD8+ T-cells may trigger keratinocyte apoptosis in OLP. Lesional T-cell clones were more cytotoxic against autologous lesional keratinocytes and normal skin keratinocytes than against autologous B-cell blasts. The majority of cytotoxic clones from lichen planus lesions were CD8+, and the majority of non-cytotoxic clones were CD4+. [15]

LICHEN PLANUS ANTIGEN

The lichen planus antigen is unknown, although the antigen may be a self-peptide, thus defining lichen planus as a true autoimmune disease. The role of autoimmunity in disease pathogenesis is supported by many autoimmune features of OLP, including disease chronicity, adult onset, female predilection, and association with other autoimmune diseases, occasional tissue-type associations, depressed immune suppressor activity in OLP patients, and the presence of auto-cytotoxic T-cell clones in lichen planus lesions.[16] Hence, an early event in lichen planus lesion formation may be keratinocyte antigen expression or unmasking at the future lesion site induced by systemic drugs (lichenoid drug reaction), contact allergens in dental restorative materials or toothpastes (contact hypersensitivity reaction), mechanical trauma (Koebner phenomenon), bacterial or viral infection, or an unidentified agent. Subsequently, intra-epithelial CD8+ cytotoxic T-cells recognize the lichen planus antigen associated with Major Histocompatibility Complex (MHC) class I on lesional keratinocytes and trigger keratinocyte apoptosis.[17]

ANTIGEN LOCATION

Controversies exist about the number and location of antigen, whether one or two antigens are involved? And Why OLP manifests at only specific site? LP has a well-defined clinical distribution and there is a clear demarcation between lesional and non-lesional tissue. A possible explanation for this pattern of presentation is that keratinocytes express the LP antigen, but only at the lesion site. In other words, the clinical distribution of lichen planus is determined by the distribution of the antigen.[18] Keratinocytes express lichen planus antigen but only at the lesion site, *i.e.*, the clinical distribution of lichen planus lesions is determined by the distribution of the lichen planus antigen. Both CD4+ T helper cells and CD8+ cytoxic T cells are activated in OLP. They are activated when presented with antigens by MHC class II and I molecules, respectively. Antigens that are presented by MHC class II are processed through an endosomal cellular pathway. In contrast, antigens that are presented by MHC class I are processed through a cytosolic cellular pathway. Hence, the putative antigen presented by MHC class II to CD4+ helper T-cells in OLP may differ from that presented by MHC class I to CD8+ cytotoxic T cells. Alternatively, a single antigen may gain access to both the endosomal and cytosolic cellular pathways of antigen presentation. For example, some viruses encode proteins that are available for cytosolic processing and expression in association with MHC class I.[19] These viral proteins are also present on the plasma membrane and therefore are available for endosomal processing and expression in association with MHC class II. In some cases of malignant transformation of OLP lesions may represent an initial lichenoid response to pre-existing tumor cells expressing elevated levels of HSP, followed by the development of overt clinical and histological malignancy. In other words OLP may not be causing malignancy directly but a response to the tumor cells.

The specific immune response to this unidentified antigen involves the following steps:
- Migration of T lymphocytes into the epithelium;
- Activation of the T-lymphocytes
- Killing of keratinocytes

Migration of T lymphocytes into the epithelium

The authors suggested that epithelial changes were initial events in disease pathogenesis. Following altered keratinocyte antigen expression, an antigen specific CD8+ T-cell may be either:-

(i) On routine surveillance in the epithelium and encounter the keratinocyte antigen by chance ("chance encounter" hypothesis) or

(ii) Attracted to the epithelium, along with T-cells of irrelevant specificity, by keratinocyte- derived chemokines ("directed migration" hypothesis).

CHANCE ENCOUNTER HYPOTHESIS -

The "chance encounter" hypothesis is supported by findings of CD8+ T-cells in normal human epidermis and basal cell degeneration in the absence of a dense inflammatory infiltrate in lichen planus lesions. The "chance encounter" hypothesis may explain the prevalence of OLP in the general population (one to two percent) and the onset of OLP in later life, *i.e.*, it takes some time for the CD8+ T-cell to encounter its specific antigen in the oral epithelium.[20]

DIRECTED MIGRATION HYPOTHESIS-

Conversely, the "directed migration" hypothesis is supported by findings of constitutive chemokine receptor expression on naive T-cells and a dermal T-cell infiltrate prior to the appearance of intra-epithelial lymphocytes and epithelial damage in lichen planus lesions.[21] In addition, pre-activation of antigen-specific CD8+ T-cells (*e.g.*, in a regional lymph node) may up-regulate inflammatory chemokine receptor expression and facilitate antigen-specific CD8+ T-cell migration to the future OLP lesion site "directed migration" hypothesis predicts that keratinocyte derived chemokines attract T-cells of irrelevant specificity along with antigen-specific T-cells into the developing OLP lesion. In support of this hypothesis, our recent studies identified a significant proportion of non-clonal OLP lesional T-cells, and not all CD8+ lesional T-cell clones were cytotoxic against autologous lesional keratinocytes .In summary, the initial event in OLP lesion formation may be keratinocyte antigen expression in association with MHC class I at the future lesion site, with or without up-regulated keratinocyte chemokine production. Pioneer antigen-specific CD8+ cytotoxic T-cells may enter the oral epithelium on routine surveillance, or they may be attracted by keratinocyte-derived chemokines. Subsequently, antigen- specific CD8+ cytotoxic T-cells trigger apoptosis of basal keratinocytes. In this context, keratinocyte antigen expression and chemokine production are primary events in OLP lesion formation, followed by keratinocyte apoptosis triggered by antigen-specific CD8+ cytotoxic T-cells. Formation of the dense subepithelial lympho-histiocytic infiltrate and epithelial basement membrane changes in OLP may result from antigen-specific interactions between keratinocytes and T-cells, or they may be epiphenomena associated with the recruitment of T cells with irrelevant specificity into the OLP lesion site. [22]

Activation of T cells

The lymphocytic infiltrate in OLP is composed almost exclusively of T cells. Binding of antigen to MHC-1 on target cell (keratinocyte) activates CD8+ cytotoxic T cell directly. MHC class II antigen presentation in OLP may be mediated by Langerhans cells (LC) or keratinocytes. There are increased numbers of LCs in OLP with up-regulated MHC Class II expression. Binding of antigen to MHC Class II present on antigen presenting cells along with secretion of Interleukin-12 activates CD4+ T helper cells. Most lymphocytes in the lamina propria are CD4+ helper T cells. They in turn activate CD8+ T cells and interleukin-2 (IL-2) and interferon-Υ (IFN-Υ) secretions. [23](Figure 3)

Killing of keratinocytes (KERATINOCYTOLYSIS)

The activated cytotoxic T cells kill the basal keratinocytes. Apoptosis has been proposed as mechanism of keratinocyte death. Cytotoxic T cell secretes Tumor necrosis factor- α (TNF-α) which triggers the keratinocyte apoptosis. [24] Possible mechanism of keratinocyte apoptosis are:
- T cell secreted TNF-α binding to TNF-α R1 receptor on keratinocyte surface.
- T cell surface CD95L (Fas ligand) binds to CD95 (FAS) on the keratinocyte surface.

- T-cell-secreted Granzyme B entering the keratinocyte via perforin induced membrane pores.

All these mechanism activate a cascade resulting in keratinocyte apoptosis. (Figure 4)

Regulation of keratinocyte apoptosis in OLP

There may be different complex pathways involved in apoptosis of basal keratinocytes, and these pathways may also have multiple interactions. FasR and FasL were highly expressed in OLP, both in the epithelium and in the subepithelial cell infiltrate and since the FasR-FasL system mediates apoptosis, it is surprising that the rate of apoptosis is rather low. This finding may indicate a functional defect in the FasR/FasL molecules or in the Fas mediated apoptotic pathway[25].

The CD40-CD40L system may play several roles in the pathogenesis of OLP, since (1) CD40 and CD40L are expressed in different cell types of OLP, and (2) multiple potential interactions of CD40/CD40L may occur with other molecules expressed in OLP. The fact that CD40-CD40L ligation may induce or inhibit apoptosis dependent on the cell type and context, further complicates the picture of the putative role of the CD40- CD40 system in the pathogenesis of OLP.

The basal keratinocytes of diseased areas in OLP may escape CD40-CD40L mediated apoptosis via down-regulation of CD40. On the other hand, the CD40 downregulation may together with the CD40L loss observed in the basement membrane zone, be a signal to promote keratinocyte renewal in areas of basal cell destruction of OLP. This suggestion is based on the fact that CD40 ligation inhibits proliferation of epidermal keratinocytes in monolayers by modulation of the cell cycle .In addition, an inverse relationship between CD40 and Ki-67, with decreased CD40 expression and increased Ki-67 expression, has been demonstrated in epidermal monolayers and normal skin biopsies. Accordingly, elevated Ki-67 expression and other proliferation markers, may support the suggestion that CD40 downregulation is a signal to promote proliferation in basal keratinocytes of OLP.[26]

Down-regulation of CD40 may also affect other apoptosis regulatory proteins including Fas and Cox-2, by interaction mechanisms. This suggestion is based on the fact that CD40 can up-regulate Fas in cancer cell lines, as well as Cox-2 on human fibroblasts and endothelial cells *in vitro*. Cox-2 has the ability to inhibit apoptosis via several pathways, as reducing both cytocrome-c and caspase activation, and up-regulation of the protooncogene Bcl-2. Consequently, the reported up-regulation of Cox-2 expression in OLP may lead to inhibition of apoptosis and thus contribute to increased cell survival. Such an anti-apoptotic effect of Cox-2 may however be disturbed by p53, due to interaction with Cox-2 as well as the ability of p53 to induce apoptosis by its own.[27] Loss of adhesive cell contacts such as E-cadherin may play specific roles in basal cell destruction of OLP. This suggestion is based on the fact that E-cadherin loss may; (1) promote apoptosis of basal keratinocytes in OLP, since reports have demonstrated that apoptosis may be prevented by E-cadherin mediated cell contact in immortalized cell lines, (2) promote T cell migration into the epithelium, where they may easier target the keratinocytes and induce apoptosis CD44 is most probably not directly involved in apoptosis of keratinocytes, since it is maintained in OLP. However, CD44 may play an indirect role in regulation of keratinocyte apoptosis in OLP by modulating other apoptosis related molecules including Fas.[28]

Taken together, apoptosis regulation is complex in OLP involving several interrelated molecules including FasR/FasL, CD40/CD40L, Cox-2, p53, CD44 and E-cadherin.

SUMMARIZING ANTIGEN SPECIFICITY IN OLP:-

> MHC class I- and MHC class II-restricted antigen presentation by lesional keratinocytes

⬇

> activation of antigen-specific CD4+ helper T-cells and CD8+ cytotoxic T-cells

⬇

> **clonal expansion of antigen-specific T-cells**

⬇

> keratinocyteapoptosis triggered by antigen-specific CD8+ cytotoxic T-cells

B. Non-Specific Mechanisms

Some of the T cells in OLP lymphocytic infiltrate are not specific. They may be attracted to and retained within OLP lesion by various mechanism associated with pre-existing inflammation which may cause destruction of keratinocytes. The various factors proposed are:

THE EPITHELIAL BASEMENT MEMBRANE

Keratinocytes contributes to the structure of the epithelial basement membrane by secreting collagen IV and laminin V into the basement membrane zone. Also keratinocyte may require a basement-membrane derived cell survival to prevent the onset of apoptosis. Thus basement membrane is required for keratinocyte survival and keratinocyte for normal basement membrane production. Apoptotic keratinocytes are no longer able to perform this function. Hence,

Keratinocyte apoptosis triggered by CD8+ cytotoxic T cells may result in epithelial basement membrane disruption in OLP which allows non-specific T lymphocytes present in subepithelial zone to migrate into the epithelium. Basement membrane disruption may trigger keratinocyte apoptosis, and apoptotic keratinocytes may unable to repair the disrupted basement membrane. Such vicious cycle may be responsible for disease chronicity.[18] (Figure 5)

MATRIX METALLOPROTEINASES

The principal function of MMPs is the proteolytic degradation of connective tissue matrix proteins. The gelatinases (*e.g.*, MMP-2 and -9) cleave collagen IV, and the stromelysins (*e.g.*, MMP-3 and -10) cleave collagen IV and laminin. MMP proteolysis is regulated by the action of endogenous inhibitors, including the tissue inhibitors of metalloproteinases (TIMPs), which form stable inactive enzyme-inhibitor complexes with MMPs or proMMPs. A higher concentration of MMP-9 was identified in patients with OLP than healthy control peripheral blood T-cells. T-cell-secreted MMP-9 may disrupt the epithelial basement membrane in OLP lesions. MMP-9-induced basement membrane disruption may facilitate the passage of antigen-specific CD8+ cytotoxic T-cells into the OLP epithelium, where they trigger further keratinocyte apoptosis.[20]

CHEMOKINES

The chemokines are a superfamily of pro-inflammatory cytokines that are produced by virtually all somatic cells. Recent studies of cutaneous lichen planus identified basal keratinocyte expression of the CC chemokine MCP-1 and two CXC chemokines MIG and IL-10. IL-8, MCP-1, and GRO gamma were expressed by IL- 1estimulated human oral keratinocytes in vitro, while oral keratinocytes from oral LP patients secreted cytokines that up-regulated mononuclear cell adhesion molecule expression and transendothelial cell migrationin vitro. These data suggest that activated keratinocytes secrete chemokines attracting lymphocytes and other immune cells into the developing oral LP lesion. Various data implicate a role for T-cell secreted regulation-upon activation, normal T expressed and secreted (RANTES) in the pathogenesis of oral LP. T cells from oral LP expressRANTES in situ. In vitro, oral LP lesional T cells expressmRNAfor RANTES and TNF-alpha stimulation up-regulates T-cell RANTES secretion. Mast cells express the CCR1 RANTES receptor in oral LP in situ. An unidentified factor in oral LP lesional T-cell supernatant, up-regulates human mast cell line (HMC-1) CCR1 mRNA expression in vitro. Oral LP lesional T-cell supernatant stimulates HMC-1 migration in vitro, while this effect is partially blocked by anti-RANTES antibody.The same supernatant stimulates HMC-1 degranulation in vitro with release of TNF-alpha and histamine. This effect is also blocked by anti-RANTES antibody.[29]

Hence, RANTES secreted by oral LP lesional T cells may attract mast cells into the developing oral LP lesion and subsequently stimulate mast cell degranulation. Degranulating mast cells release TNF-alpha, which upregulates T-cell RANTES secretion. Such a cyclical mechanism may promote disease chronicity. Furthermore, RANTES induces expression of PI 3-kinase, which is involved in signal transduction for both chemotaxis and mitogen-activated protein kinase activation. PI 3-kinase activates Akt/protein kinase B that is an important component of the cell's prosurvival machinery. Both T cells and mast cells express CCR1 in oral LP. Hence, in addition to stimulating mast-cell chemotaxis and degranulation, RANTES secreted by lesional T cells may also prolong the survival of inflammatory cells in oral LP and thereby contribute to disease chronicity.

MAST CELLS

Studies showed increased mast cell density in OLP and hence proposed to be involved in the pathogenesis.[28] Their results showed that degranulated mast cells had a higher cell count in OLP lesion hence proposed to be involved in the pathogenesis. Mast cell degranulation in OLP releases a range of pro-inflammatory mediators such as TNF-a, Chymase, and Tryptase. TNF-a may up-regulate endothelial cell adhesion molecule (CD62E, CD54, and CD106) expression in OLP that is required for lymphocyte adhesion to the luminal surfaces of blood vessels and subsequent extravasation. It also stimulates RANTES secretion by lesional T cells. Chymase is a known activator of MMP-9 which causes basement membrane disruption in OLP. Both TNF-α and Chymase stimulate secretion of RANTES by T lymphocytes which in turn stimulate mast cells to release TNF-α and Chymase.[18, 28] (Figure 6)

SUMMARIZING NON-SPECIFIC MECHNISMS IN OLP:-

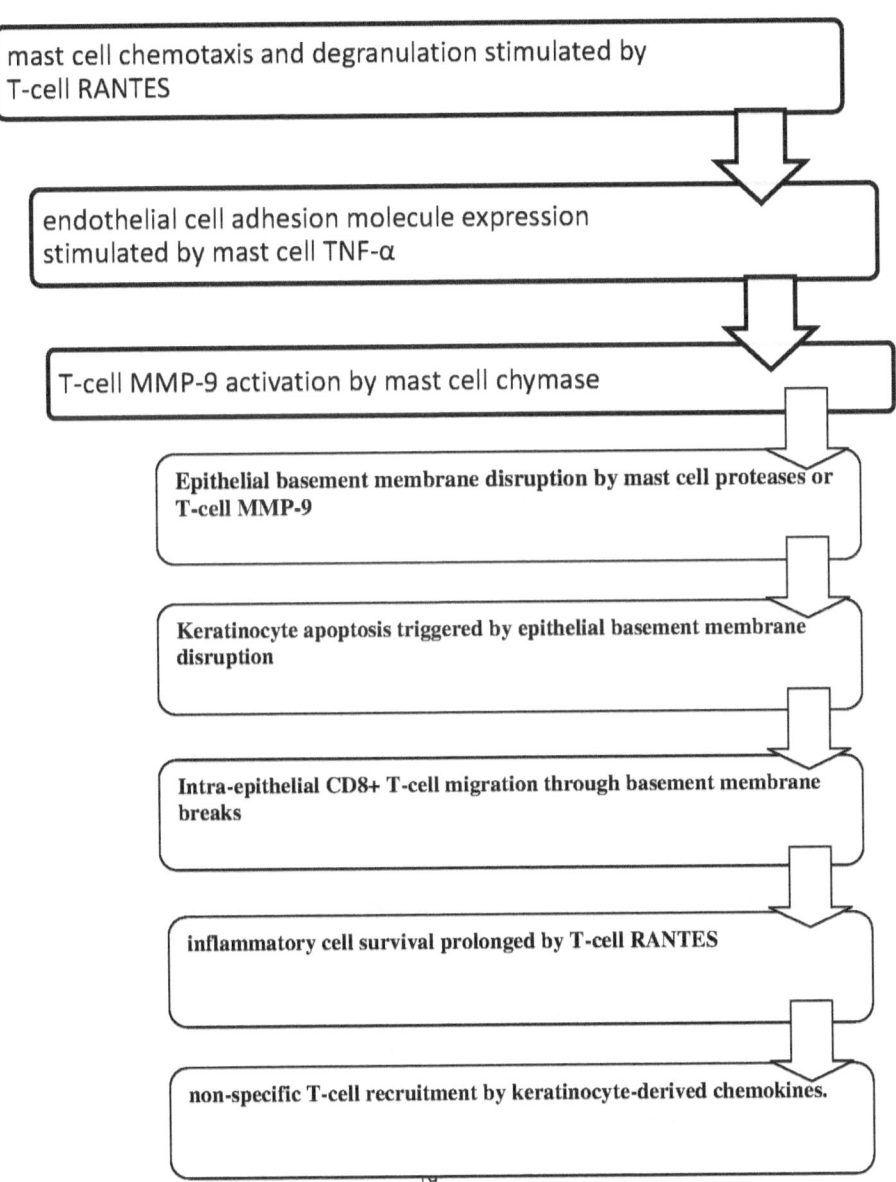

C. AUTOIMMUNITY

OLP is hypothesized to be an autoimmune disease. The role of autoimmunity in disease pathogenesis is supported by many other autoimmune features of OLP including, disease chronicity, adult onset, female predilection, association with other autoimmune diseases, occasional tissue type associations, depressed immune suppressor activity in OLP and auto-cytotoxic T cell clones in OLP. Four hypotheses have been proposed implicating autoimmune reaction in OLP. They are:-

- Deficient antigen-specific immune-suppression in OLP- lack of TGF-β1
- Breakdown of immune privilege in OLP
- Keratinocyte apoptosis and langerhans cell maturation in OLP.
- Heat Shock Protein

Deficient antigen-specific immune-suppression in OLP- lack of TGF-β1

TGF-β1 has immunosuppressive effects. Weak expression of TGF- β1 has been found in OLP which may predispose an auto-immune lymphocytic inflammation. OLP chronicity may be part of it. TGF-b1 immunosuppressive pathway involving:-

(i)   insufficient numbers of TGF-b1-secreting Th3 regulatory T-cells,

(ii) blockage of TGF-b1 secretion

(iii) secretion of non-functional TGF-b1,

(iv) Defective or inadequate TGF-b1 receptor expression,

(v)   Defective intracellular signaling downstream from the TGF-b1 receptors.

The balance between TGF-b1 and IFN-g signaling may determine the level of immunological activity in OLP lesions.[11, 14, 15]

Breakdown of immune privilege in OLP

OLP may result from a failure of resident keratinocytes to trigger T-cell apoptosis. Oral keratinocytes in OLP may fail to express enough active TNF-α, or the release of TNF-α from the surfaces of oral keratinocytes in OLP may be blocked, possibly due to defective MMP activity. (Figure 7)

The normal oral mucosa may be an immune privileged site, similar to the eye, testis, and placenta. In the eye and testis, immune privilege is mediated by Fas ligand (CD95L), expressed by stromal cells that triggers apoptosis of infiltrating inflammatory cells expressing Fas (CD95). This mechanism is thought to minimize potentially damaging inflammation in these organs. A similar mechanism (oral keratinocyte CD95L or TNF-a triggering T-cell apoptosis *via* CD95 or TNF R1, respectively) may prevent excessive T-cell infiltration in the normal oral mucosa, while failure of such a mechanism may result in OLP and possibly other autoimmune oral mucosal diseases, including cicatricial pemphigoid and pemphigus vulgaris.[11, 14] (Figure 7)

Keratinocyte apoptosis and langerhans cell maturation in OLP

To stimulate a T-cell response, dendritic cells (DCs) and presumably LCs must undergo a process of terminal differentiation called "maturation". Stimuli for DC and LC maturation include inflammatory cytokines (IL-1b, TNF-a), CD40L (CD154) expressed by activated T-cells, necrotic cells, HSPs, nucleotides, reactive oxygen intermediates, neurotransmitters, MMP-9, extracellular matrix degradation products, mechanical trauma, various allergens, ion channel blockade, Fc receptor aggregation, viral RNA, and bacterial lipopolysaccharide.

Under normal circumstances, APCs carrying selfpeptides derived from apoptotic cells do not receive a maturation stimulus and therefore do not trigger an auto-reactive T-cell response. Immature APCs may avoid activating self-reactive T-cells by various means, including

(i)   failure to form MHC-peptide complexes,

(ii)   absence of co-stimulatory molecule expression, or

(iii)   direct killing of self-reactive T-cells

Conversely, APC endocytosis of apoptotic cells followed by APC maturation may activate self-reactive CD4+ T-cells that differentiate into Th1 or Th2 phenotypes and promote cell- or antibody-mediated autoimmune reactions. The nature of the APC maturation stimulus (*e.g.*, cytokines, CD40L, necrotic cells, HSPs, etc.) may determine the outcome (Th1 *vs.* Th2) of CD4+ T-cell activation.[11, 14] (Figure 8)

Heat Shock Protein

Heat shock proteins form an ancient, primary system for "intracellular self-defense". They are highly conserved class of protective cellular proteins that are produced under various conditions of environmental challenge. They have been implicated as the antigen stimulus in autoimmune diseases. Most of the heat shock proteins are molecular chaperones. Chaperones have been defined as "proteins that bind to and stabilize an otherwise unstable conformer of another protein – and, by controlled binding and release, facilitate its correct fate *in vivo*: be it folding, oligomeric assembly, transport to a particular subcellular compartment, or disposal by degradation"[30]

Heat shock proteins (Hsp) are induced by a large variety of stimuli besides heat shock itself.[31] (Table 1)

Heat shock	Too much Ca ions inside the cell
Cold shock	Viral infection
UV radiation	Bacterial products
Electro smog	Parasite toxins
Amino acid analogues	Acute phase reaction
Alcohol	Overload of Endoplasmic reticulum
Heavy metal ions	Phaghocytosis
Arsenite	Hormonal effects
Too much oxidation	Increased cell proliferation
Too much reduction	Cell differentiation
Too little glucose	Increased blood pressure
Too little ATP	Too little exercise
Feeding of cell cultures	Too much exercise
Osmotic Shock	Mental stress

Table 1

Heat shock proteins play an essential role in the etiology of numerous diseases, with a rapidly increasing role in clinical practice. Their function is necessary for the homeostasis of the living cell, and becomes especially important in disease, when our cells have to cope with a stressful environment. Molecular chaperones are one of the most conserved proteins in living organisms.

Invading bacteria experience major changes in their environment when entering their host. These changes and the activation of defense mechanisms (depletion of nutrients, pH changes, osmotic changes, digestive enzymes, peroxides, superoxides and an increase in temperature) induce numerous heat shock proteins in bacteria, among which some are also expressed on the bacterial surface. Because of their conservative structure, these bacterial heat shock proteins, especially the bacterial homologue of Hsp70 become a common recognition signal, and therefore provoke a general, high-capacity immune response. There are at least two dozen infectious diseases in which immune responses to heat shock porteins have been reported, including tuberculosis, leprosy, legionnaire's disease, Chagas's disease, lyme disease, chlamidyal infections and Q fever. In some unfortunate cases (such as in rheumatoid arthritis, in lupus erythematosus, in multiple sclerosis and in insulin dependent diabetes mellitus, IDDM) certain proteins of the host organism resemble some epitopes of these bacterial heat shock proteins. In these patients the common, antibacterial immune response attacks the cells bearing these host-proteins, and a severe autoimmune response develops. Vaccination with modified epitopes of a bacterial Hsp70 homologue diminishes, and in some cases prevents the development of the disease. Some recent reports raise the possibility that expression of human Hsp60 on the surface of epithelial cells may be one of the initial events of arterial plaque development.[30, 31]

Hsp is found to be elevated in OLP. T cell immune reaction to keratinocyte Hsps (or cross reaction to bacterial Hsps) remains as a possible mechanism for the development and persistence of LP.[32] Hsp70 and Hsp90 as well as their counterparts in the endoplasmic reticulum, such as Grp94, give each other the peptides and help their presentation to the MHC-I complex, specialized to present the "self" antigens to the immune system. MHC-I molecules induce a cytotoxic T-cell response, which is a fast and local immune attack, against a cell expressing "false" self-antigens (e.g. after a viral infection). This may significantly enhance the efficiency of the MHC-II immune response, which is based on helper T lymphocytes, and generates a slow and general immune attack.[30, 31]

D HUMORAL IMMUNITY

There is currently little definitive evidence to implicate an altered humoral immune response in the pathogenesis of OLP. OLP has rarely been associated with hypogammaglobulinanemia. Association of OLP with autoimmune diseases has been well documented but the frequency of autoimmune diseases observed in large group of OLP patients is not always elevated in comparision with the general population. There is no significantly raised frequency of the autoimmune-associated HLA antigens B8, DR3, or DR4 in OLP. Moreover, OLP patients exhibit no consistant alteration in the serum level of immunoglobulins. Varried levels of IgA, IgG, IgM and IgD have been observed in OLP with no change in serum components.[11]

Within lesional and perilesional tissue of idiopathic OLP there is no consistent or pathogonomic deposition of immunoglobulins, fibrinogen or complement components. IgM may present at basement membrane zone. IgM are found on collid bodies. IgA and IgG may occasionally present. A lichen planus specific antigen (LPSA) in granular or spinous layer has been described; however it has been inconsistently present in affected patients although patients may have antibodies to LPSA. Recently, another autoantibody to keratinocytes have been described, and immunoglobulin deposits have been demonstrated at the basement membrane zone of OLP patients with lichenoid reactions which may not be specific to lichenoid reaction and if OLP does have an autoimmune basis, it is more likely to involve cell-mediated immune reactions rather than aspects of humoral immunity.[33]

OTHER POSSIBLE MECHANISMS OF PATHOGENESIS OF LICHEN PLANUS

Mechanism similar to Chronic Graft Vs Host disease

Graft-versus-host disease (GVHD) is a common serious complication following allogeneic hematopoietic stem cell transplantation (HSCT), and is a major cause of HSCT-related mortality. Acute GVHD occurs within the first 100 days of transplantation and comprises dermatitis, enteritis, and by viral infection, bacterial products, mechanical trauma, systemic drugs, contact sensitivity or an unidentified agent. Activated APCs and keratinocytes secrete chemokines that attract lymphocytes into the developing oral LP lesion. Activated APCs present antigen associated with MHC class II to CD41 T cells. Activated basal keratinocytes present antigen associated with MHC class I to CD81 T cells (2b). CD40 and CD80 coexpression and IL-12 secretion by MHC class II1 APCs promotes a T helper-1 (Th1) CD41 T-cell response. Th1 CD41 helper T cells secrete IL-2 and IFN-gamma (3a), which bind their respective receptors onCD81 T cells (3b). Activated antigen-specific CD81 cytotoxic T cells express FasL or secrete granzyme B or TNF-alpha that trigger basal keratinocyte apoptosis.[14]

Chronic GVHD develops after day 100 and comprises an autoimmune-like syndrome comparable to ulcerative colitis, primary biliary cirrhosis, Sjö"gren's syndrome, rheumatoid arthritis, and lupus-like disease with glomerulonephritis. The skin is a primary target in chronic GVHD and exhibits either a lichenoid eruption or sclerodermatous changes. Oral involvement occurs in 33% to 75% of patients with acute GVHD and up to 80% of patients with chronic GVHD.Oral mucosal GVHD resembles oral LP both clinically and histologically. As with oral LP, squamous cell carcinoma (SCC) may develop in oral and cutaneous chronic GVHD.[15]

Most patients who undergo allogeneic HSCT receive stem cells from MHC-identical donors. In these patients, GVHD is initiated by donor T cells that recognize a subset of host peptides called minor histocompatibility antigens (miHAs). Although the antigen specificity of LP and mucocutaneous GVHD is probably distinct, it is likely that they share similar immunological effector mechanisms resulting in T-cell infiltration, epithelial basement membrane disruption, basal keratinocyte apoptosis, and clinical disease. Hence, research findings in one disease may give clues to the pathophysiology of the other. The role of TNF-alpha as a major effector molecule in GVHD has been confirmed in a number of experimental systems. Importantly, neutralizing anti-TNF-alpha antibodies have been shown to alleviate cutaneous and intestinal GVHD in both mice and humans. Blockade of the CD40-CD154 costimulatory pathway prevented GVHD following allogeneic HSCT. The role of the Fas apoptotic pathway in cutaneous GVHD is less clear. In one study, the transfer of cells lacking Fas-L (CD95L) reduced the severity of murine cutaneous GVHD. In another study, recipient mice deficient in Fas (CD95) showed increased severity of cutaneous GVHD. An MMP inhibitor was shown recently to alleviate GVHD pathology in the liver, intestine, and hematopoietic tissues and reduce weight loss and mortality in murine GVHD.[14, 15]

To further elucidate the cellular and molecular mechanisms of lichenoid cutaneous pathology, a recent study correlated detailed histopathology with global gene expression in a murine model of cutaneous GVHD. Cutaneous GVHD was induced by MHC matched allogeneic HSCT, and ear skin was examined at days 7, 14, 21, and 40 post-transplantation. On day 7 post-HSCT, the skin appeared relatively normal with the only pathological changes consisting of rare dermal vessels cuffed by occasional lymphocytes and dermal mast cells containing clear cytoplasmic vacuoles indicating degranulation. By day 14, lymphocytes were diffusely present within the dermis and focally within the epidermal layer in association with early keratinocyte apoptosis. Gene expression patterns were consistent with early infiltration and activation of

CD81 T and mast cells, followed by CD41 T, natural killer (NK), and myeloid cells. The sequential infiltration and activation of effector cells was accompanied by upregulated expression of many chemokines and their receptors (CXCL1, 2, 9, 10; CCL2, 5, 6, 7, 8, 9, 11, 19; CCR1, CCR5), adhesion molecules (ICAM-1, CD18, Ly69, PSGL-1, VCAM-1), molecules involved in antigen processing and presentation (TAP1 and 2, MHC class I and II, CD80), regulators of apoptosis (granzyme B, caspase 7, Bak1, Bax, and Bcl2), and interferon-inducible genes (STAT1, IRF-1, IIGP, GTPI, IGTP, Ifi202A). On day 14 and thereafter, the epidermal thickness exceeded twice that observed on day 7, and the superficial epidermis exhibited marked hypergranulosis. These observations correlated with up-regulated expression of keratins 5 and 6 (markers of keratinocyte proliferation) and small proline-rich proteins 2E and 1B (markers of keratinocyte differentiation). By days 21 and 40 post-HSCT, there were multiple foci of epidermal apoptosis and the entire dermal thickness was more than twice that observed on days 7 and 14. The latter observation was associated with up-regulated expression of IL-1b and TGF-b1 that stimulate fibroblast proliferation and matrix synthesis.[34]

Many acute phase proteins were up-regulated early in murine cutaneous GVHD including serum amyloid A2 (SAA2), SAA3, serpins a3g and a3n, secretory leukocyte protease inhibitor, and metallothioneins 1 and 2. These intriguing gene expression findings in murine cutaneous GVHD are currently under investigation in oral LP.

ANGIOGENESIS

Angiogenesis represents a cycle of vital processes that leads to the neoformation of anomalous blood vessels in pre-existing vascular structures. At the heart of angiogenesis is the endothelial cell that proliferates and differentiates under the regulatory action of vascular endothelial growth factor (VEGF), the principal direct inducer of angiogenesis together with other growth cofactors. This process plays an important role both in physiological conditions, such as embryonic development and the healing of wounds, and in pathological conditions, such as the growth of tumours and metastasis and the development of chronic inflammatory diseases. Scientific studies have shown the importance of angiogenesis in the chronic inflammatory mechanism and have verified the presence of neoangiogenesis in pathologies.

Recently role of Angiogenesis is studied in oral lichen planus.[35] It has found to play role in other autoimmune disorders such as rheumatoid arthritis, psoriasis, bronchial asthma, diabetic retinopathy, atherosclerosis and Alzheimer's disease. Furthermore, recent studies have confirmed a strong involvement of the angiogenetic phenomenon in other intestinal chronic inflammatory diseases such as Crohn's Disease and ulcerous rectocolitis. It is known that angiogenesis plays a key role in the pathogenesis of chronic inflammatory illnesses, not only causing the gemmation of new vessels that allow a better oxygenation and a greater contribution of metabolites to the proliferating tissue, but also notably increasing the complex system of feed-back and turnover of the cells involved in the inflammatory process. This feed-back mechanism has been noticed the presence - in isolated endothelial cells - of the prominent factor in the angiogenetic phenomenon: VEGF.[35]

Oral lichen planus (OLP) is a pathology of the oral mucous of a chronic inflammatory autoimmune pathogenetic mechanism in which a rich vascular proliferation has been seen, probably as a reaction to the hypoxic effect on the stromal area, where the phlogistic reaction occurs due to the increase of proliferating lymphocytes. The markers VEGF, CD34, VCAM-1 and ICAM-1 are appropriate to investigate the vascular endothelin and they have been used in the study to probe the presence of angiogenesis process and to underline endothelial modifications. The literature is not, at the moment, satisfactory and up-to-date compared with the study of the angiogenetic phenomenon in OLP. As an autoimmune disease with an inflammatory origin and chronic progression, OLP satisfies all the prerequisites of hypoxia at the base of the angiogenetic mechanism in light of the hypoxic effect caused by the proliferating inflammatory elements that has also been found in the oral mucous with nonhistological or serological techniques, such as videocapillaroscopy. Studies affected on patients affected by OLP have had as their point of interest the increase of the number of mastocytes up to the level of the lamina itself. Such studies have proved how such an increase of density can, in effect, influence the vascular endothelia in a critical way and have an important role in the formation phase of the lesion. Immunohistochemical studies performed in the past have suggested that there is the intervention of the angiogenetic phenomenon in the malignant transformation of a lot of precancerous lesions of the oral epithelium, including OLP, but such studies were hypothetical and aimed at the oncologic consequence of the lesion.

The assessment of the expression of the inducer factors of angiogenesis represents an important departure point for the study of new therapies based on the use of antiangiogenetic medicines already used in other pathologies with chronic inflammatory pathogenesis with good results. Moreover, the verified presence of angiogenesis in OLP could give further clarifications with respect to the ethiopathogenesis of OLP, which is still unknown today. In conclusion, the individualization of both lymphocytes in transit among the cubic endothelial cells of the neoformed vessels and adhesion molecules (anti-VCAM-1 and anti-ICAM-1antibodies) in the endothelial cells of such vessels, suggests that angiogenesis in the lichen not only restores tissue oxygenation but also develops an important role in the turnover of the inflammatory elements in the inflamed area and therefore in the self-perpetuation of the disease. (Figure 10)

CHANGES IN THE EXPRESSION OF STEM CELL MARKERS IN ORAL LICHEN PLANUS AND HYPERKERATOTIC LESIONS

Despite the pivotel role of stem cells in homeostasis of oral epithelial, the location of this cell population within the tissue is uncertain. How disease influences these cells in vivo also remains to be elucidated.

Kose et al in 2007 in a study showed the location of stem cells in normal non-keratinised buccal epithelium (NOM) by immunohistochemical staining for the putative stem cell markers alpha 6 and beta 1 integrins, melanoma-associated chondroitin sulphate proteoglycan (MCSP), NG2 the rat homologue of human MCSP, notch 1 and keratin 15 (k15).[36] This is the first study to show alterations in stem cell marker expression in oral lichen planus & oral hyperkeratotic lesions which indicates pathological signaling may regulate expression of these markers. This implicates adult stem cells in the pathogenesis of these mucosal disorders where epithelial differentiation and proliferation is known to be perturbed. k15, NG2 and beta 1 staining was continuous in the basal layer of NOM whilst α 6 and β 1 and MCSP were up-regulated in both OLP & OHK. NG2 remained unchanged & notch 1 was absent in all samples. Therefore, the stem cell phenotype in OLP and OHK may be altered in response to pathological signaling. Classification of these changes is essential to understand the role of adult stem cells in the pathogenesis of oral diseases characterized by abnormal keratinocyte proliferation and differentiation.

Staining pattern observed in the study showed that α 6 integrin and MCSP are the most likely adult stem cell markers in oral epithelium. High expression of the integrin family of receptors is believed to be responsible for stem cells being more adhesive to basement membrane than other basal cells. Further studies of these molecular perturbations are essential to understand the fundamental role of adult stem cells in the pathogenesis of benign mucosal disease.

A UNIFYING HYPOTHESIS FOR THE PATHOGENESIS OF OLP

Lichen planus antigen is expressed in association with MHC class I molecules on keratinocytes at the OLP lesion site. Antigen-specific CD8+ cytotoxic T-lymphocytes (CTLs) are activated in the OLP epithelium (possibly with help from Th1 CD4+ T-cells, as discussed previously) and trigger keratinocyte apoptosis *via* secreted TNF-a, although roles for granzyme B and Rantase cannot be excluded at this stage. TNF-a may be activated and released from the CTL surface by lesional MMPs. Activated T-cells undergo intra-lesional clonal expansion and release RANTES and other cytokines that up-regulate mast cell CCR1 expression and stimulate intra-lesional mast cell migration and degranulation . Degranulating mast cells release TNF-α, which up-regulates endothelial cell adhesion molecule expression for lymphocyte adhesion and extravasation. Mast cell TNF-a also up-regulates RANTES and MMP-9 secretion by OLP lesional T-cells. Activated lesional T-cells (and possibly keratinocytes) secrete chemokines which attract extravasated lymphocytes toward the OLP epithelium. Degranulating mast cells release chymase that damages the epithelial basement membrane directly or indirectly *via* activation of MMP-9 secreted by OLP lesional T-cells. Epithelial basement membrane disruption facilitates the passage of lymphocytes into the OLP epithelium and denies keratinocytes a cell survival signal, resulting in further keratinocyte apoptosis.[14] (Figure 11)

PRECIPITATING FACTORS FOR OLP/OLR

As previously mentioned, OLP is unlikely to be caused by a single antigen. In a minority of patients, precipitating factors have been identified, including infectious agents dental materials, drugs, stress ETC [37] (Table 2)

List of causative/exacerbation factors of OLP/OLR
Drugs
Anti malarial
Non-Steroidal Anti-inflammatory Drugs (NSAID)
ACE Inhibitors
Diuritics
Beta Blockers
Oral Hypoglycemics
Gold salts
Penicillamine
Anti-retroviral
Dental Materials
Dental Amalgam
Composite and Resin based materials
Metals (nickel)
Chronic Liver Disease/ Hepatitis C
Stress
Genetics
Tobacco Chewing
Graft Vs host disease

Table 1

1. **Infectious Agents**

Among the exogenous factors, several infective agents including some viruses and Helicobacter pylori have recently been linked withoral LP but sometimes on the basis of equivocal data[38].

Herpes viruses

Almost all the 8 recognized human herpesviruses may give rise to oral lesions and 4 (Herpes simplex 1[HSV-1], Epstein-Barr virus [EBV], Cytomegalovirus [CMV], Herpes virus 6 [HHV-6]) have been implicated in oral LP. DNA from HSV-1,CMV, and HHV-6 has occasionally been found within oral LP tissue, mainly in erosive lesions and in small series. However, there are no significant differences in the prevalence of both immunoglobulin (Ig)G and IgM antibodies to CMV or HHV-6 between oral LP patients and controls. The receptor for EBV (CD21) is up-regulated in oral LP and a significantly higher optometric density of EBV anti-earlier antigen (EA) IgG positivity has been reported in oral LP compared with controls, despite no difference in the frequency of both EBV IgG and IgM for EA and nuclear antigen-1 (EBNA) but it is unclear if EBV may be involved in the pathogenesis or is secondary to the oral LP lesions. [15, 38]

Human Immunodeficiency Virus (HIV)

A few cases have been reported of lichenoid lesions in patients with HIV infection, but most of them could be related to zidovudine or ketaconazole therapy.[15, 39]

Human papillomavirus (HPV)

Human papillomaviruses (HPV) are small epitheliotropic DNA viruses that can induce hyperplastic, papillomatous, and verrucous squamous cell lesions in the stratified squamous epithelia. Studies to detect different HPV types in various oral mucosal diseases have been limited or have involved a small number of samples. It is extremely difficult to compare results because of the many differences in inclusion criteria, clinical features (erosive vs nonerosive lesions), sampling of material (biopsies or brushing), preparation methods (fresh, frozen, or fixed), geographic differences, and methods adopted. Since highly sensitive techniques such as PCR may cause false-positive reactions, positive results in the literature should be viewed with caution. In fact, detection of HPV-DNA does not prove a casual relationship, since its presence in the lesional tissue may be casual or result from the disease process or immunosuppressive therapy, as shown by a recent case report of HPV reactivation following treatment of penile erosive LP.[15, 39, 40] (Table 3)

Country	Reference	Detection of HPV in OLP %	Technique	HPV probe used	Specimen positive for that genotype
Finland	Syrjanen et al 1986	2/2 (100)	ISH	6,11,16	6(1),16(1)
United kingdom	Maitland et al 1987	7/8 (87.5)	SBH	1,2,4,6,11,13,18	16(6)
USA	Kashima et al 1990	0/21 (0)	ISH	6,11,16,18,31	
Sweden	Jontell et al 1990	6/20 (65)	SBH	6,11,16,18	11(6)

Sweden	Jontell et al 1990	13/20 (65)	PCR	6,11,16,18	6(5),11(8),16(3)
USA	Young et al 1991	0/6 (0)	ISH	6,11,16,18,31,33,35	
USA	Miller et al 1993	0/8(0)	ISH	6,11,16,18,31,33,35,24,43, 44,45,51,52,56	
United kingdom	Cox et al 1993	2/4 (50)	SBH	16	16(2)
Germany	Vesper et al 1997	3/7 (42)	PCR	NA	NA
Spain	Gonzalez-Moles et al 1998	2/17 (11.8)	PCR	16	16(2)
Sweden	Sand et al 2000	6/22 (27.3)	PCR	NA	NA
Itlay	Giovannelli et al 2002	9/34 (26.5)	PCR	NA	NA

Table 1. ISH, in situ hybridization; SBH, southern blot hybridization; PCR, polimerase chain reactions; NA, not available.

Hepatitis viruses

It was first reported by Mokni et al in 1991.[41] The frequent association of LP with chronic liver disease (CLD) is well-known, especially in Mediterranean patients with oral erosive LP, but no hypothetical pathogenic correlation could be found until sensitive hepatitis C virus (HCV) assays became available.

An association between OLP and HCV has been reported in literature. The two main hypotheses regarding the mechanism of HCV induced OLP are that[5]:

    a. HCV may replicate within the oral epithelium, thus directly contributing to development of OLP lesions.

    b. HCV is a virus that has a high rate of mutation which results in the repeated activation of immune cells, increasing the likelihood of cross reaction with self tissue and therefore heightening the risk of developing autoimmune diseases.

The frequent association of LP with chronic liver disease (CLD) is well documented, at least in Mediterranean patients with oral LP, whereas prospective studies of Scandinavian and British oral LP patients have failed to show any significant correlation with liver diseases. The role of particular HCV genotypes in the pathogenesis of HCV-related OLP is ruled out by the observation that LP can be associated world-wide with the same genotypes commonly found in patients without LP, though mainly genotype 1b seems associated with LP, and it appears to be uncommon in the UK.[5]

Interestingly, geographic heterogeneity in the prevalence of HCV infection similar to that observed in OLP patients was also found in patients with other extrahepatic abnormalities linked to HCV infection, such as serum autoantibodies, porphyriacutanea tarda (PCT), and lymphoma The major histocompatibility complex (MHC) class II alleles was found to influence the geographic heterogeneity of the association between oral lichen planus (OLP) and hepatitis C virus infection (HCV). Specific major MHC class II alleles may influence susceptibility (HLA-DRB1*0701, HLA-DRB4*0101) or resistance (HLA-DRB1*1101, HLA-DQB1*0301) to persistent HCV infection.[42] (Table 3)

Country	Reference	LP (n)	HCV+ %	Serological test	HCV-RNA %
Brazil	Issa et al 1999	34	5.9	Unspecified	NA
	Figueiredo et al 2002	68	8.8	ELISA 2	NA
Egypt	Ibrahim et al 1999	43	20.9	Unspecified	NA
France	Cribier et al 1994	52	3.8	ELISA+RIBA2	NA
	Dupin et al 1997	102	4.9	ELISA+RIBA3	NA
Germany	Imhof et al 1997	83	16	ELISA+RIBA2	14
Italy	Rebora 1994	56	23	Unspecified	NA
	Carrozzo 1996	70	27.1	ELISA+RIBA2	21.4
	Serpico et al 1997	100	32	ELISA+RIBA2	NA
	Mignobna et al 1998	263	28.8	ELISA+RIBA2	NA
Japan	Tanei et al 1995	45	37.8	ELISA 2	NA
Nepal	Garg et al 2002	86	0	ELISA 3	NA
Nigeria	Daramola et al 2002	57	15.8	ELISA 2	NA
Spain	Gimenez-Arnau et al 1995	25	44	Unspecified	NA
	Sanchez-Perez et al 1996	78	20	ELISA 2	16
	Bagan et al 1998	100	23	ELISA+RIBA2,3	NA
	Glimenez-Garcia et al 2003	101	8.9	ELISA+RIBA2	NA
Turkey	Ilter et al 1998	72	0	Unspecified	NA

	Kirtak et al 2000	73	6.8	ELISA 3	NA
	Erkek et al 2001	54	12.9	ELISA 3	9.3
United Kingdom	Ingafou et al 1998	55	0	ELISA 3	NA
	Tucker et al 1999	45	0	ELISA+RIBA2,3	NA
USA	Bellman et al 1995	30	23	ELISA+RIBA2	16
	Chuang et al 1999	22	55	ELISA 2	NA
	Beaird et al 2001	24	17	Unspecified	NA

Table 4 NA-not available

2. Dental Restorative materials

supposed to cause OLP/OLL including amalgam, composite, resin, cobalt and gold. Mainly amalgam has been deeply studied as a possible triggering factor. Some authors suggested that sensitization to mercury (main component of amalgam) is an important cause that these lesion might represent a delayed hypersensitivity response to mercury. Dental material in direct contact to oral mucosa may directly alter the antigenicity of basal keratinocytes by release of mercury and other products. Contact allergy to dental material mostly involve delayed type IV hypersensitivity reaction which involve cell mediated immunity mainly T lymphocytes and macrophages which are sensitized to antigen. However in some studies removal may not always prove to be beneficial which suggests involvement of other factors. An alternate explanation to lesion related to restoration may be an immunological and toxin reaction to plaque accumulation over surface of restoration and such lesion may disappear after improvement of oral hygiene. [12, 37]

3. Drugs and Medications

Systemic medications such as anti malarial drugs, non-steroidal anti-inflammatory agents (NSAIDs), angiotensin converting enzyme inhibitors (ACE inhibitors), Beta Blokers, Penicillamin may induce OLP/OLL. Other drugs reported to cause OLP/OLR are diuritics, gold salts, oral hypoglycemic and recently anti-retroviral drugs for treatment of human immunodeficiency virus (HIV) infection have been reported to cause OLP/OLR. [12, 37]

4. Stress

Exacerbation of OLP may be linked to period of physiological stress and anxiety. Burkhart NW et al concluded that there is relationship between stress and oral lichen planus.[7] Heat shock proteins (Hsps) also known as stress protein was found to be up regulated in OLP. There are psychologic alterations in OLP patients which is either a direct cause of the disease or a consequence of OLP. Rojo-Moreno JL et al Levels of anxiety are raised in the OLP patients and found that there are psychologic alterations in OLP patients which may be either a direct cause of the disease or a consequence of OLP. [43] Rodstrom PO et al concluded that there is no impaired capacity of OLP patients to suppress an immune response through cortisol induction in conjunction with stress.[44] Ivanovski K et al however, supported that cortisol and psychological status may play a role in the pathogenesis of OLP, especially in the erosive form of the disease but the findings need to be replicated in larger study population that includes males also.[45] Moreover, major drawback of these studies were that no other predisposing factors of OLP has been estimated in patients due to which authors cannot conclude that whether psychologic alterations in OLP patients is either a direct cause of the disease or a consequence of OLP.

5. Genetics.

Several studies have proposed to show an association between HLA antigens and OLP. The frequency of HLA-DR1 is found to be increased in patients with OLP. The frequency of HLA-DRw9 was found to be significantly raised in Japnese patients and also in group of Chinese patients. HLA-B27, HLA-B51 and HLA-Bw57 has been found in a group of English patients with OLP whereas, HLA-DR2 in Israeli Jewish patients.[5]

The recent consistent observation of increase in HLA-DR suggests being involved in the pathogenesis of OLP.[46, 47]

Montebugnoli L et al concluded that genetic instability found in some patients should be interpreted as a consequence of the enhanced epithelial turnover.[48] Tao XA et al found that concluded that the gene expression profile of patient with OLP is quite distinct from that of healthy controls.[49] Yarom N et al also supported that OLP carries an increased risk for chromosomal instability.[50]

NEW PROSPECTIVE TO THE UNDERSTANDING OF OLP

We tried to explore every aspect of lichen planus (LP) and found that it is complicated to identify a single etiologic factor behind its pathogenesis. Various precipitating factor discussed earlier altogether makes the etiology behind LP to be a multifactorial process comprising events that may take place at different time points. Analysis of data clearly suggests OLP to be a chronic inflammatory reaction as described by many authors earlier which includes migration of T lymphocytes particularly CD8+ cells and CD4+ along with mast cells at the OLP site leading to keratinocyte apoptosis. These T cells are found to be activated by an antigen. Due to presence of clusters of CD8+ T cells in the basal epithelial layer in the region of basement membrane disruption it can be said the lichen planus antigen can be presented by MCH class I molecules which is present on all cells. However, due to presence of CD4+ T cells in epithelium and lamina propria of OLP lesion it is arguable that lichen planus antigen can also be presented by MCH class II molecules present mostly in the membrane of the antigen presenting cells (dendritic and phagocytic cells). Single antigen may gain access to be presented by both the MHC molecules. For example, some viruses encode proteins that are available for cytosolic processing and expression in association with MHC class I. These viral proteins are also present on the plasma membrane and therefore are available for endosomal processing and expression in association with MHC class II. This suggests that antigen can be more than one.

Question still remains that how and when does OLP initiate and what are these antigens which causes oral lichen planus? When cell is under stress due to many causes including heavy metal ions, viral and bacterial products, hormonal effects, increased blood pressure, mental stress, etc. it induces an ancient and primary system for intracellular self defense known as "Heat

Shock Proteins" (Hsp) which is actually beneficial to the body. It binds to an otherwise unstable conformer of another protein and facilitates its correct fate i.e. folding, transport to particular sub cellular compartment or disposal by degradation. Invading bacteria or virus experiences major changes in their environment when entering their host. These changes and the activation of defense mechanisms (depletion of nutrients, pH changes, osmotic changes, digestive enzymes, peroxides and rise in temperature) induces numerous Hsp in bacteria among which some are also expressed on the bacterial surface. In some unfortunate cases (such as in rheumatoid arthritis, in lupus erythematosus, in multiple sclerosis and in insulin dependent diabetes mellitus, IDDM) certain proteins of the host organism resemble some epitopes of these bacterial heat shock proteins. In these patients the common, antibacterial immune response attacks the cells bearing these host-proteins, and a severe autoimmune response develops. Similar alteration of proteins may be caused by dental restorative materials, drugs or by mechanical trauma causing alteration of proteins at the site or restoration leading to an immune response over the site which causes keratinocyte apoptosis.

Why only keratinocytes expresses LP antigen? This may be due to role of genetic in the pathogenesis of the disease. The lesional keratinocyte may present Human Leukocyte Antigen (HLA-DR) antigens on their surface, which may have an inductive or perpetuating role in initiating the cellular reaction. It has been well estimated by various authors that HLA-DR may be responsible for the peculiar geographic heterogeneity of association between HCV and OLP. So it can be concluded that HLA-DR allele makes a patient more susceptible to OLP. But viral infection of the oral mucosa produces a T-cell response that typically does not progress to OLP. Mechanical trauma to the oral mucosa causes mast cell degranulation that typically does not progress to OLP. Similarly all patients possessing HLA-DR allele do not progress to OLP. So, what constitutes OLP susceptibility? Answer to this question can be a combination of factors, including deregulated oral keratinocyte antigen expression, persistence of mature oral LCs, circulating auto-reactive T-cells, and defective immune suppressor activity following self-antigen recognition which also accounts for OLP being a multifactorial disease in which different precipitating factors play role at different point of time.

There have been numerous studies quoting a positive relationship between psychological stress and OLP. A major drawback of these studies was that the authors were unable to conclude that whether psychologic alterations in OLP patients are either a direct cause of the disease or a consequence of OLP.

A long controversy has been associated with OLP; weather is an autoimmune reaction or a chronic inflammatory immune response. Factors which supports OLP being an autoimmune disease are:-

- Chronicity
- Adult onset
- Female predilection
- Association with other autoimmune diseases
- Occasional tissue type associations
- Depressed immune suppressor activity
- Auto-cytotoxic T cell clones

Factors which do not support OLP being an autoimmune disease are:-

   o OLP is not known to be associated with autoimmune disease.

- o No generalized involvement of body
- o T cells are over responsive in over one site.

We proposed OLP to be a chronic inflammatory reaction appearing as an autoimmune disease.

Our unifying hypothesis for pathogenesis of OLP is that both antigen-specific and non-specific mechanisms are involved in oral lichen planus (OLP). Antigen-specific mechanisms in OLP include antigen presentation by basal keratinocytes and antigen-specific keratinocyte killing by CD8+ cytotoxic T-cells. Non-specific mechanisms include mast cell degranulation and matrix metalloproteinase (MMP) activation in OLP lesions. Chemokines like RANTES plays a crutial role in recruitement of lymphocytes, monocytes, natural killer cells, eosinophils, basophils and mast cells. Mast cells in OLP would release TNF-α and chymase which in turn regulate OLP lesional T-cell RANTES secretion.

These mechanisms may combine to cause T-cell accumulation in the superficial lamina propria, basement membrane disruption, intra-epithelial T-cell migration, and keratinocyte apoptosis in OLP. Apoptotic cell death of epithelial keratinocytes is complex, and a number of biological changes that may induce or inhibit apoptosis are found in the basal cell compartment of OLP compared to normal OM.

- Basal keratinocytes die by apoptosis in OLP. Apoptosis is increased in areas with basal cell destruction and regions with atrophic epithelium in OLP. Apoptosis may be dysregulated in the subepithelial mononuclear cell infiltrate, contributing to maintenance of the massive inflammatory cell infiltrates in OLP.

- There may be a dysfunction in the FasR-FasL mediated apoptosis in keratinocytes and T cells of OLP.
- Basal keratinocytes may escape a CD40-CD40L mediated apoptotic mechanism in OLP by down-regulation of CD40 in diseased areas.
- Cox-2 is widely expressed and up-regulated in OLP, and may inhibit apoptosis of keratinocytes.
- E-cadherin loss in basal keratinocytes may promote apoptosis and contribute to basal cell destruction, allowing T cell migration into the epithelial compartment in OLP.

OLP chronicity may be due, in part, to deficient antigen-specific TGF-b1-mediated immunosuppression. The normal oral mucosa may be an immune privileged site (similar to the eye, testis, and placenta), and breakdown of immune privilege could result in OLP and possibly other autoimmune oral mucosal diseases. Recent findings in mucocutaneous graft-*versus*-host disease, a clinical and histological correlate of lichen planus, suggest the involvement of TNF-a, CD40, Fas, MMPs, and mast cell degranulation in disease pathogenesis. Carcinogenesis in OLP may be regulated by the integrated signal from various tumor inhibitors (TGF-b1, TNFa, and IFN-g IFN C g-12) and promoters (MIF, MMP-9).

IS ORAL LICHEN PLANUS IS A PRE-MALIGNANT DISEASE?

One of the biggest controversy in understanding of OLP is that is OLP is premalignant? No significant co-relation has been found with its association with smoking or alcohol. Frequency of malignant transformation ranges from 0.4% to 10%.[51] nactivation of p53 is a frequent phenomenon in OSCC. This is caused by mutations, presence of HPV virus and other molecular alteration occurring in the p53 pathway [52]. The studies investigating the expression of p53 in OLP have been recently reviewed by Ebrahimi et al. [53]. In their vast majority, they included immunohistochemistry-based reports and their results varied significantly, with reported expression percentages ranging from 0–100%. Nevertheless, most of them found significantly higher expression in OLP than in normal oral mucosa [53]. As p53 expression has been identified as a response to DNA damage, [54]the identification of p53 in OLP tissue is interpreted as an indication of precancerous potential by some researchers[55]. In support to this concept, Chaiyarit et al. showed an i-NOS-dependent DNA damage and p53 elevated expression in OLP patients [56]. Another concept is that the high expression of p53 in OLP is a result of the higher cellular proliferation [57]. To prove that p53 expression in OLP is not just a result of the inflammatory process, Safadi et al. [55] compared the immunohistochemical expression of p53 and of its downstream effector p21^{WAF1} between OLP and other inflammatory oral conditions and found significantly higher expression in OLP [38]. What is still unclear is the underlying mechanism that drives p53 expression in a significant percentage of OLP cases, but as p53 expression in OLP is comparable to that observed in dysplastic oral lesions, it is considered as a sign of malignant potential.

At this point, it is tempting to speculate that OLP as an inflammatory condition, along with the accompanying oxidative stress, probably induces a genotoxic stress. In addition, the high proliferation rates reported for the oral epithelium turnover in OLP may also create a replication stress. Such conditions should activate the DNA damage response (DDR) checkpoint [58, 59]. In turn, this pathway should elicit the p53-mediated antitumor barriers of apoptosis and senescence. Continuous activation of this checkpoint will eventually surpass the cell repair capacity predicting the emergence of genomic instability and finally selective p53 inactivation. Consecutively, this would result in the progression to malignancy. Nevertheless, this scenario requires experimental validation, despite the presence of experimental evidence compatible with it.

Chromosomal Instability in OLP

To verify the OLP malignant potential hypothesis, genetic alterations observed in epithelial cancers have also been studied in OLP. In 1997, Zhang et al. used microsatellite analysis to investigate loss of heterozygosity (LOH) at loci 3p, 9p, and 17p, which is frequently observed in oral cancers [60]. Despite they detected LOH, their results showed no different frequencies from the reactive irritation (benign inflammation). Nevertheless, while this result did not support OLP as a lesion at risk for malignant transformation, the authors could not exclude that OLP may undergo malignant transformation through other genetic pathways [61]. Following these results, the same authors performed the same loci analysis in dysplastic lesions in OLP patients and their results showed comparable rates of allelic loss with those observed in epithelial dysplasia even for cases of mild dysplasia [62]. From this finding they concluded that dysplasia observed in OLP cases is possibly an independent risk factor for malignant transformation and underlined that very diligent clinical and pathologic approach should be applied in the case of OLP biopsies [62]. Similar results and conclusions especially for LOH in chromosome 9 in OLP-associated dysplasia were reported by Kim et al. with the use of chromosomal *in situ* hybridization [63]. On the other hand, in a more recent study using laser capture microdissection and microsatellite analysis to identify LOH, the results were similar in benign lesions and OLP samples weakening the concept of malignant OLP potential, but these authors also emphasize on careful histopathologic examination of OLP samples [64]. Of note, all data available from LOH analyses are confined only to chromosomes 3, 9, and 17 [60-63]. To the best of our knowledge, genome-wide analyses in large cohorts of OLP are still missing.

Changes in DNA ploidy are also an indication of malignancy. DNA ploidy studies in OLP have demonstrated that some atrophic lesions may be found aneuploid, but the results are not indicative of a potentially malignant process [64-66]. Abnormal karyotypes and chromosomal alterations associated with p53 expression have also been detected in OLP, but the data are small to allow safe conclusions [67].

DETAILED ASPECTS OF TREATMENT

Various treatments have been employed to treat symptomatic oral lichen planus, but complete resolution is difficult to achieve.[68] summarizes treatment options for oral lichen planus. Topical corticosteroids are first-line therapy.[69-71] High-potency topical steroids are the most effective, with response rates up to 75 percent compared with placebo.[72] Topical corticosteroids are also first-line therapy for mucosal erosive lichen planus.[69] High-potency corticosteroids applied to the oral mucosa do not appear to cause significant adrenal suppression, even with relatively long-term use. Systemic corticosteroids, such as oral prednisone, should be considered only for severe, widespread oral lichen planus and for lichen planus involving other mucocutaneous sites.[73]

Topical calcineurin inhibitors, such as tacrolimus and pimecrolimus (Elidel), are second-line therapies for oral lichen planus.[74] A comparative study showed that topical tacrolimus is as effective as the high-potency corticosteroid clobetasol in the treatment of oral lichen planus.[74] A randomized controlled trial revealed that pimecrolimus 1% cream effectively treats erosive oral lichen planus with long-lasting therapeutic effects.[75]

In a randomized controlled trial, aloe vera gel was significantly more effective than placebo in the clinical and symptomatologic improvement of oral lichen planus.[76] If topical corticosteroids are ineffective, carbon-dioxide laser evaporation can lead to long-term remission of symptoms, and may be appropriate as first-line therapy in patients with painful oral lichen planus.

THERAPEUTIC APPROACH BASED ON THE NEW CONCEPT

While exploring the cause of a disease we can use a linear model for causation. But many diseases are multi-factorial with multiple risk factors. This is usually explained as "Web of Causation" theory of disease. However while analyzing factors associated with OLP, we find that there are conflicting and confusing results. The typical confluence of factors causing the disease cannot be validated in OLP. Diverse causes have been found to have a significantly strong association with OLP like Stress, hormonal imbalance, heavy metal ions, viral products, increased blood pressure, drugs, human leucocyte antigen (HLA) gene, etc but only in small fraction of the cases of OLP. Hence, based on the new prospective towards the pathogenesis of the disease several therapeutic approaches may be considered for OLP following its pathogenesis like:

1. Antibodies to TNF-α and interferons-Υ
2. Stabilization of mast cells to prevent degranulation
3. Vaccine which alter the false presenting self peptide into true one.
4. Immunosuppressive medications which alter adhesion molecule expression and impair lymphocyte function may be of benefit.
5. Potential use of agents such as interleukin-8, TGF-β and interleukin-1 inhibitors which reduces leukocyte trafficking thereby reducing chronicity of disease.

CONCLUSION

The modern view of etiology and pathogenesis of most of the diseases suggest them to be influenced by multiple factors, hence requiring a simultaneous evaluation of factors concerned with various areas. This concept holds true for oral lichen planus. The pathogenesis of OLP may involve both antigen-specific and non-specific mechanisms. Antigen-specific mechanisms in OLP include antigen presentation by basal keratinocytes and antigen-specific keratinocyte killing by CD8+ cytotoxic T-cells. Nonspecific mechanisms include mast cell degranulation and matrix metalloproteinase activation in OLP lesions. The initial event in OLP lesion formation and the factors that determine OLP susceptibility are unknown.

Many questions remain concerning the etiology and pathogenesis of OLP. Most of them have been answered by our vast search during our research. But still some questions needs to be answered like what is the lichen planus antigen? Does the lichen planus antigen vary from site to site or patient to patient? What proportion of T-cells in OLP lesions is specific for the lichen planus antigen? Answers to these questions may help produce a cure for OLP. In the meantime, analysis of current data suggests that blocking IL-12, IFN-g, TNF-a, RANTES, or MMP-9 activity or up-regulating TGF-b1 activity in OLP may be therapeutic.

Clearly, more work is required for a full understanding of the etiology and pathogenesis of OLP.

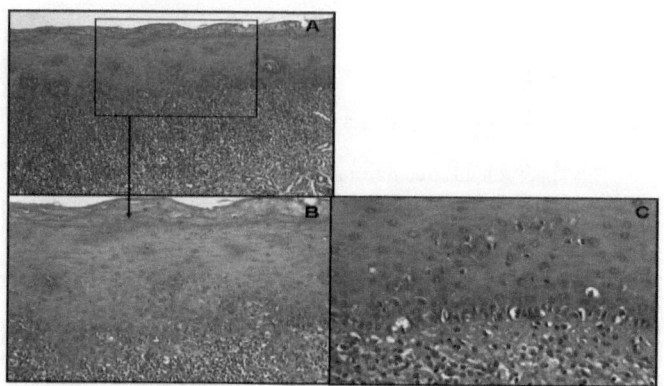

Figure 1. Oral lichen planus with subepithelial chronic inflammatory cell infiltrate (**A**), destruction of the basal cell layer (**B**) and cell death of basal keratinocytes (**C**). Hematoxylin & Eosin. Orig. magn: x100 (A), x200 (B), x400 (C).

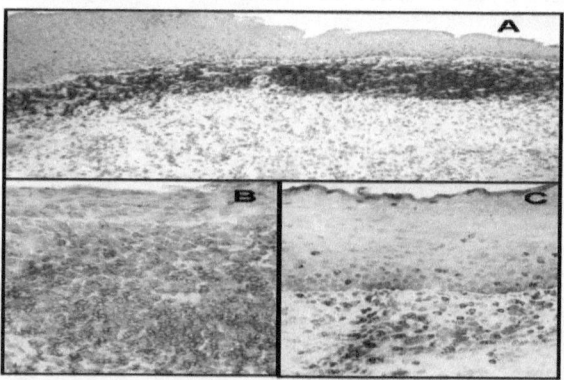

Figure 2 CD3+ (**A**) CD4+ (**B**) and CD8+ cells (**C**) in the epithelium and subepithelial cell infiltrate of oral lichen planus. Immunohistochemistry. Orig. magn: x100 (A) x250 (B, C).

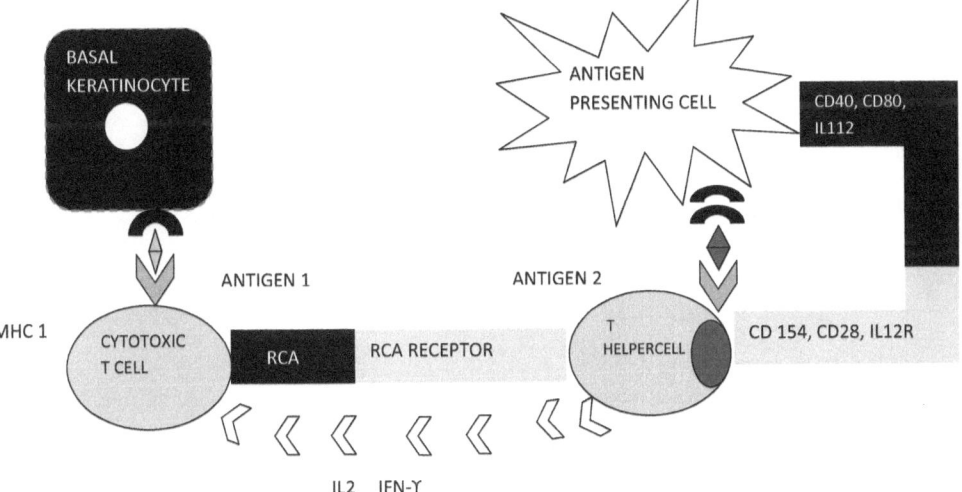

Figure 3. Activation of cytotoxic T cells by antigen presented by MHC I on basal keratinocyte, activation of T helper cells from antigen presented by Langerhans cells and In turn activation of cytotoxic T cells by Interleukin 2 and interferon gamma request for cytotoxic activity (RCA) receptors.

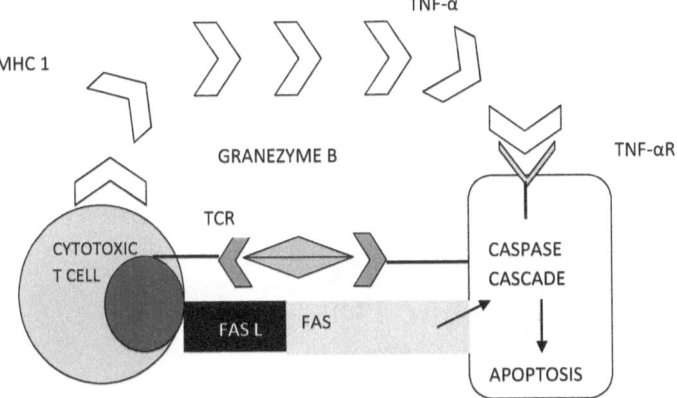

Figure 4. Mechanism of apoptosis of basal keratinocyte BASAL KERATINOCYTE nd interactions between basal keratinocyte and cytotoxic T cells, Production of Granenzyme B by cytotoxic cells and tumor necrosis factor (TNF-α) from cytotoxic T cell binding to its receptor on keratinocyte.

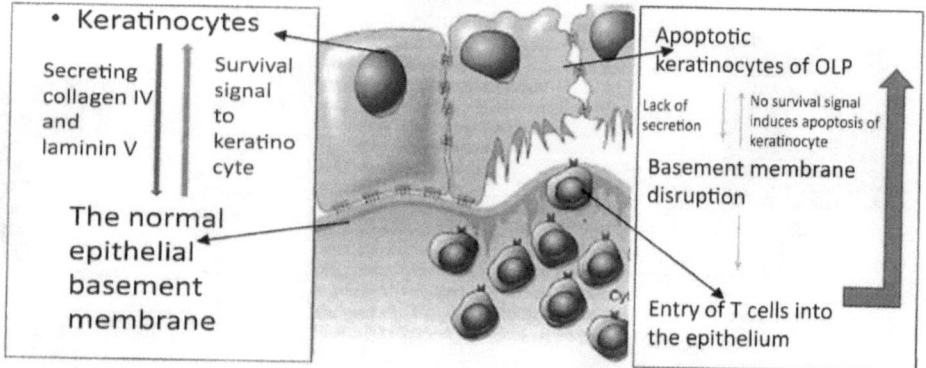

Figure 5. Role of basement membrane in keratinocyte survival is shown on the left side. The right side shows the consequences of basement membrane disruption resulting in keratinocyte apoptosis and T cell migration into epithelium

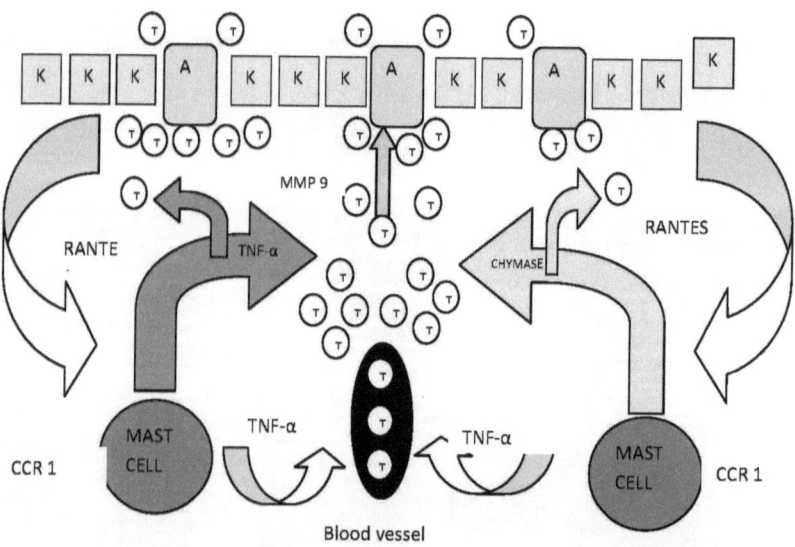

Figure 6. Role of Mast cells in the pathogenesis of LP. TNF-α are secreted by mast cell. TNF-α stimulates extravasations of T lymphocytes (T) from blood vessels. T cell release pro-MMP9 which activates MMP9 causing disruption of basement membrane. TNF and chymase stimulate

T cells to produce RANTES which further activates mast cell CCR1 receptors and stimulates degranulation. K- Basal keratinocyte A- Apoptotic keratinocytes.

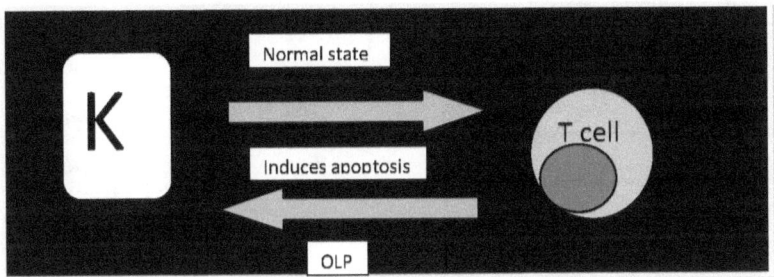

Figure 7. Keratinocyte induces apoptosis of T cells in normal state. In OLP, T cells induces apoptosis of keratinocyte.

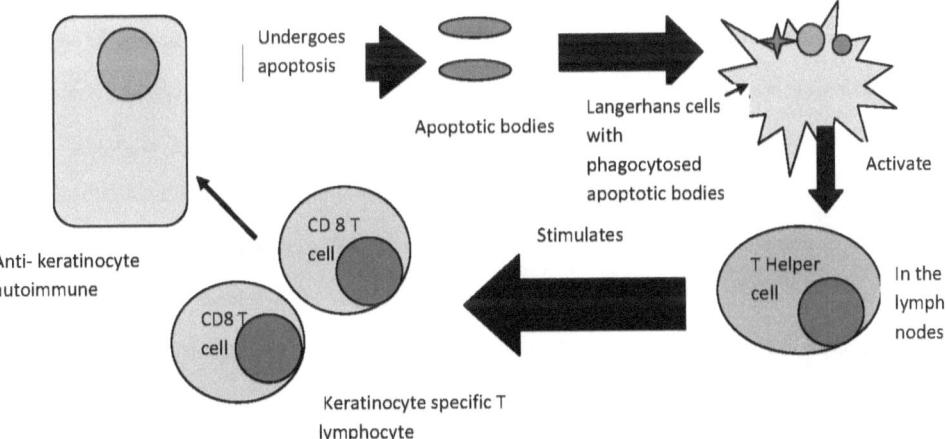

Figure 8. Mechanism of anti keratinocyte autoimmune reaction. Langerhans cells phagocytose the apoptotic bodies from basal keratinocytes and present it to T helper cells which inturn stimulates cytotoxic T cells against basal keratinocyte.

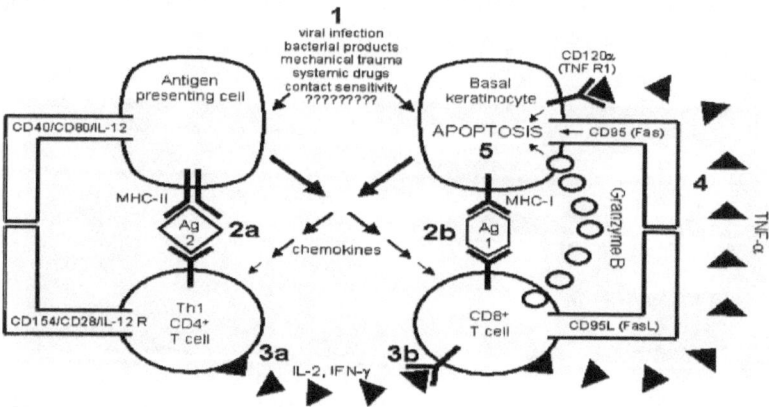

Figure 9 Hypothesis for the immunopathogenesis of oral LP. Antigen presenting cells (APCs) and basal keratinocytes are "activated" by viral infection, bacterial products, mechanical trauma, systemic drugs, contact sensitivity or an unidentified agent (1). Activated APCs and keratinocytes secrete chemokine that attract lymphocytes into the developing oral LP lesion. Activated APCs present antigen associated with MHC class II to CD41 T cells (2a). Activated basal keratinocytes present antigen associated with MHC class I to CD81 T cells (2b). CD40 and CD80 co expression and IL-12 secretion by MHC class II1 APCs promotes a T helper-1 (Th1) CD41 T-cell response. Th1 CD41 helper T cells secrete IL-2 and IFN-gamma (3a), which bind their respective receptors on CD81 T cells (3b). Activated antigen-specific CD81 cytotoxic T cells express FasL or secrete granzyme B or TNF-alpha (4) that trigger basal keratinocyte apoptosis (5).

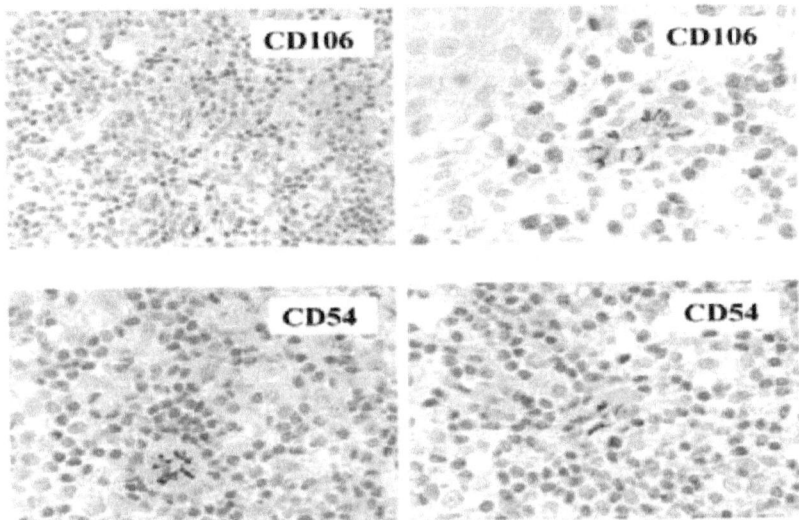

Figure 10 Oral Lichen Planus: positivity of vessels neoformed to CD106 and CD54 antibodies cells (magnification 40X).

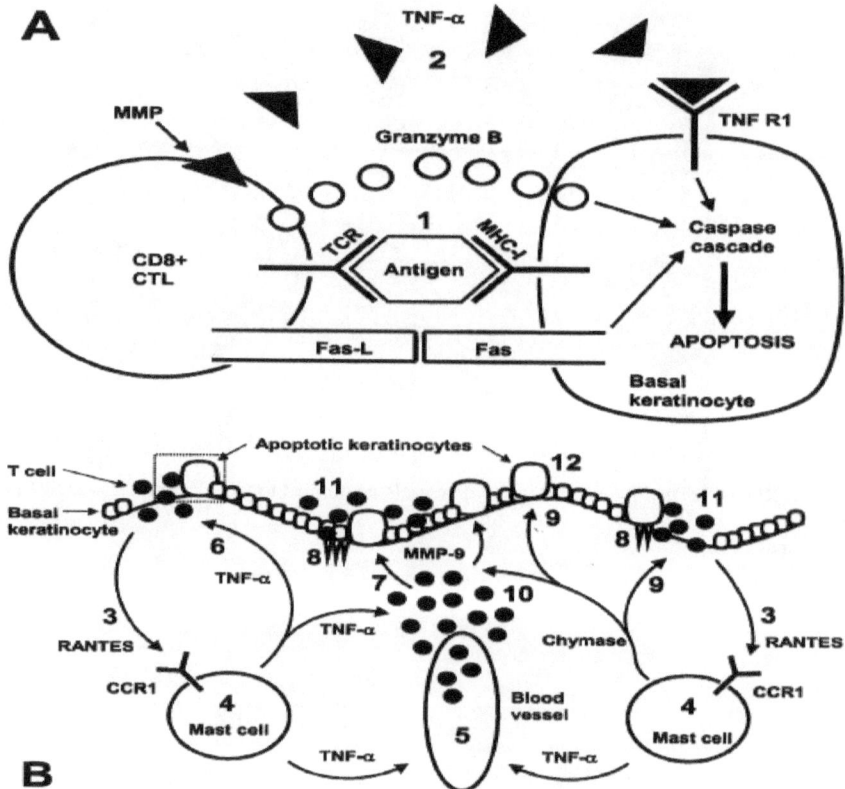

Figure 11. Unifying hypothesis for the pathogenesis of OLP. (A) A lichen planus antigen is expressed in association with MHC class I molecules on basal keratinocytes at the OLP lesion site [1]. Antigen-specific CD8+ cytotoxic T-lymphocytes (CTLs) are activated in the OLP epithelium (possibly with help from Th1 CD4+ T-cells, as shown in Fig. 1) and trigger keratinocyte apoptosis *via* secreted TNF-a binding the TNF-a receptor (TNF-R1) [2], although roles for granzyme B and Fas cannot be excluded at this stage. TNF-a may be activated and released from the CTL surface by lesional MMPs. (B) Activated T-cells undergo intra-lesional

clonal expansion and release RANTES and other cytokines [3] that up-regulate mast cell CCR1 expression and stimulate intra-lesional mast cell migration and degranulation [4]. Degranulating mast cells release TNFa, which up-regulates endothelial cell adhesion molecule expression for lymphocyte adhesion and extravasation [5]. Mast cell TNF-a also upregulates RANTES [6] and MMP-9 [7] secretion by OLP lesional T-cells. Activated lesional T-cells (and possibly keratinocytes) secrete chemokines that attract extravasated lymphocytes toward the OLP epithelium [8]. Degranulating mast cells release chymase that damages the epithelial basement membrane directly [9] or indirectly *via* activation of MMP-9 secreted by OLP lesional T-cells [10]. Epithelial basement membrane disruption facilitates the passage of lymphocytes into the OLP epithelium [11] and denies keratinocytes a cell survival signal, resulting in further keratinocyte apoptosis [12]. (A) Represents the boxed area in (B).

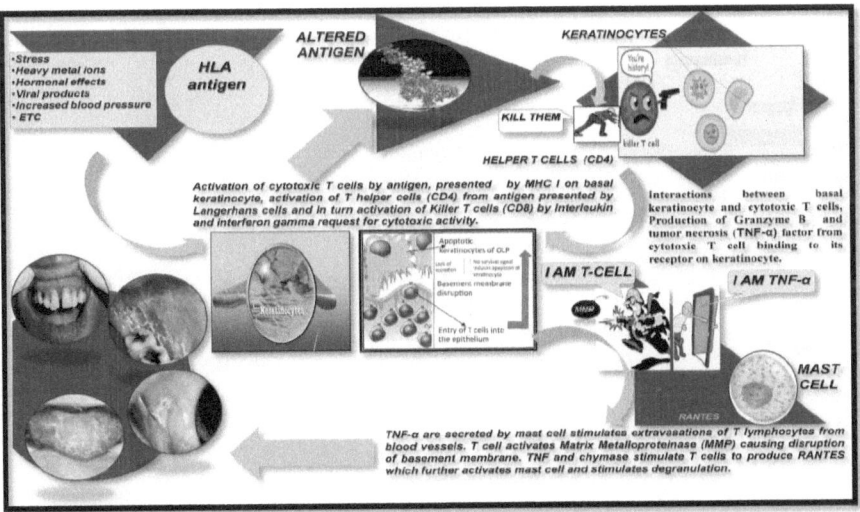

Figure 12: Simple pictorial presentation of proposed pathogenesis of Oral Lichen Planus

ABBREVIATIONS

FasL	Fas ligand
FasR	Fas receptor
LP	Lichen planus
NF-κB	Nuclear factor kappa B
OLP	Oral lichen planus
OM	Oral mucosa
OSCC	Oral squamous cell carcinoma
TNF	Tumor necrosis factor
TNFR	Tumor necrosis factor receptor
TRAF	TNF receptor associated factor
ELISA	Enzyme linked Immunosorbant Assay
PCR	Polymeric Chain Reavtion
Hsp	Heat Shock Protein

REFERENCES

1. Prado RF, Marocchio LS, Felipini RC. Oral lichen planus versus oral lichenoid reaction: difficulties in the diagnosis. . Indian J Dent Res. 2009 Jul-Sep; 20(3):361-4.

2. Greenberg MS, Glick M, Ship JA. BurKet's Oral Medicine (Eleventh edition) ; 2008

3. Aghahosseini F, Arbabi-Kalati F, Fashtami LA, Mohsen F, Djavid GE. Treatment of oral lichen planus with photodynamic therapy mediated methylene blue:A case report. Med Oral Patol Oral Cir Bucal 2006;11:E126-9

4. Neville BW, Damm DD, Allen CM, Bouquot JE. Oral and Maxillofacial Pathology (Second edition) ; 2002

5. Chainani-Wu N, Lozada-Nur F, Terrault N. Hepatitis C virus and lichen planus: a review. Oral Surg Oral Med Oral Pathol Oral Radiol Endod. 2004 Aug; 98(2):171-83.

6. Yildirim B, Sengiiven B, Demir C. Prevalence of herpes simplex, Epstein Barr and human papilloma viruses in oral lichen planus. Med oral Patol Oral Cir Bucal.20011 Mar 16 (2):170

7. Burkhart NW, Burker EJ, Burkes EJ, Wolfe L. Assessing the characteristics of patients with oral lichen planus. J Am Dent Assoc. 1996 May; 127(5): 655-6

8. Carrozzo M, Brancatello F, Dametto E, Arduino P, Pentenero M, Rendine S, Porter SR, Lodi G, Scully C, Gandolfo S. Hepatitis C virus-associated oral lichen planus: is the geographical heterogeneity related to HLA-DR6? J Oral Pathol Med. 2005 Apr; 34(4):204-8.

9. Porter SR, Kirby A, Olsen I, Barrett W. Immunologic aspects of dermal and oral lichen planus: a review. Oral Surg Oral Med Oral Pathol Oral Radiol Endod. 1997 Mar; 83(3):358-66.

10. Yarom N, Shani T, Amariglio N, Taicher S, Kaplan I, Vered M, Rechavi G, Trakhtenbrot L, Hirshberg A. Chromosomal numerical aberrations in oral lichen planus. J Dent Res. 2009 May; 88(5):427-32.

11. Roopashree MR, Gondhalekar RV, Shashikanth MC, George J, Thippeswamy SH, Shukla A. Pathogenesis of oral lichen planus--a review. J Oral Pathol Med. 2010 Nov; 39(10):729-34.

12. Carrozzo M, Thorpe R. Oral lichen planus: a review. Minerva Stomatol. 2009 Oct; 58(10):519-37.

13. Mollaoglu N. Oral lichen planus: a review. Br J Oral Maxillofac Surg 2000; 38: 370-377

14. Sugerman PB, Savage NW, Walsh LJ, Zhao ZZ, Zhou XJ, Khan A, Seymour GJ, Bigby M. The pathogenesis of oral lichen planus. Crit Rev Oral Biol Med. 2002; 13(4):350-65.

15. Zhou XJ, Sugerman PB, Savage NW, Walsh LJ, Seymour GJ. Intra-epithelial CD8+ T cells and basement membrane disruption in oral lichen planus. J Oral Pathol Med. 2002 Jan; 31(1):23-7.

16. Jahanshahi G, Aminzadeh A. A histochemical and immunohistochemical study of mast cells in differentiating oral lichen planus from oral lichenoid reactions. Quintessence Int. 2010 Mar; 41(3):221-7.

17. Farthing PM, Cruchley AT. Expression of MHC class II antigens (HLA DR, DP and DQ) by keratinocytes in oral lichen planus. J Oral Pathol Med. 1989 May; 18(5):305-9.

18. Valsecchi R, Bontempelli M, Rossi A, Bellavita P, Barcella A, Di Landro A, Cainelli T. HLA-DR and DQ antigens in lichen planus. Acta Derm Venereol. 1988; 68(1):77-80.

19. Guyton AC, Hall JE. Textbook of Medical Physiology (Eleventh edition) ; 2006

20. Bos JD, Zonneveld I, Das PK, Kreig SR, van der Loos CM, Kapsenberg ML. The skin immune system (SIS): Distribution and immunophenotype of lymphocyte subpopulations in normal human skin. J Invest Dermatol 1987; 88:569-73.

21. Spetz A-L, Strominger J, Groh-Spies V. T cell subsets in normal human epidermis. Am J Pathol 1996; 149:665-74.

22. Liu GX, Xie Q, Zhou CJ, Zhang XY, Ma BL, Wang CQ, Wei FC, Qu X, Sun SZ. The Possible Roles of OPN-Regulated CEACAM1 Expression in Promoting the Survival of Activated T Cells and the Apoptosis of Oral Keratinocytes in Oral Lichen Planus Patients. J Clin Immunol. 2011; Jun 14

23. Yamamoto T, Nakane T, Osaki T. The mechanism of mononuclear cell infiltration in oral lichen planus: the role of cytokines released from keratinocytes. J Clin Immunol 2000; 20:294-305.

24. Thongprasom K, Dhanuthai K, Sarideechaigul W, Chaiyarit P, Chaimusig M. Expression of TNF-alpha in oral lichen planus treated with fluocinolone acetonide 0.1%. J Oral Pathol Med. 2006 Mar; 35(3):161-6.

25. Hadzi-Mihailovic M, Raybaud H, Monteil R, Jankovic L. Expression of Fas/FasL in patients with oral lichen planus. J BUON. 2009 Jul-Sep;14(3):487-93.

26. Neppelberg E, Loro LL, Oijordsbakken G, Johannessen AC. Altered CD40 and E-cadherin expression--putative role in oral lichen planus. J Oral Pathol Med. 2007 Mar; 36(3):153-60.

27. Lysitsa S, Samson J, Gerber-Wicht C, Lang U, Lombardi T. COX-2 expression in oral lichen planus. Dermatology. 2008; 217(2):150-5.

28. Ebrahimi M, Boldrup L, Wahlin YB, Coates PJ, Nylander K. Decreased expression of the p63 related proteins beta-catenin, E-cadherin and EGFR in oral lichen planus. Oral Oncol. 2008 Jul;44(7):634-8.

29. Iijima W, Ohtani H, Nakayama T, Sugawara Y, Sato E, Nagura H, Yoshie O, Sasano T. Infiltrating CD8+ T cells in oral lichen planus predominantly express CCR5 and CXCR3 and carry respective chemokine ligands RANTES/CCL5 and IP-10/CXCL10 in their cytolytic granules: a potential self-recruiting mechanism. Am J Pathol. 2003 Jul; 163(1):261-8.

30. Feige, U., Morimoto, R.I., Yahara, I. and Polla, B. (eds., 1996) Stress Inducible Cellular Responses, EXS vol. 77, Birkhauser Verlag, Basel.

31. Welch, W.J. (1992) Mammalian stress response: Cell physiology, structure/function of stress proteins, and implications for medicine and disease. Physiol. Rev. 72, 1063–81.

32. Bramanti TE, Dekker NP, Lozada-Nur F, Sauk JJ, Regezi JA. Heat shock (stress) proteins and gamma delta T lymphocytes in oral lichen planus. Oral Surg Oral Med Oral Pathol Oral Radiol Endod. 1995 Dec; 80(6):698-704.

33. Walsh LJ, Savage NW, Ishii T, Seymour GJ. Immunopathogenesis of oral lichen planus. J Oral Pathol Med. 1990 Oct; 19(9):389-96.

34. Pimentel VN, de Matos LS, Soares TC, Adam R, Metze K, Correa ME, de Souza CA, Cintra ML. Perforin and granzyme B involvement in oral lesions of lichen planus and chronic GVHD. J Oral Pathol Med. 2010 Nov; 39(10):741-6.

35. Scardina GA, Ruggieri A, Messina P, Maresi E. Angiogenesis of oral lichen planus: a possible pathogenetic mechanism. Med Oral Patol Oral Cir Bucal. 2009 Nov 1; 14(11):e558-62.

36. Köse O, Lalli A, Kutulola AO, Odell EW, Waseem A. Changes in the expression of stem cell markers in oral lichen planus and hyperkeratotic lesions. J Oral Sci. 2007 Jun; 49(2):133-9.

37. G, Scully C, Carrozzo M, Griffiths M, Sugerman PB, Thongprasom K. Current controversies in oral lichen planus: report of an international consensus meeting. Part 2. Clinical management and malignant transformation. Oral Surg Oral Med Oral Pathol Oral Radiol Endod. 2005 Aug; 100(2):164-78.

38. Shimoyama T, Horie N, Kato T, Kaneko T, Komiyama K. Helicobacter pylori in oral ulcerations. J Oral Sci. 2000 Dec; 42(4):225-9.

39. Schiødt M. Less common oral lesions associated with HIV infection: prevalence and classification. Oral Dis. 1997 May; 3 Suppl 1:S208-13.

40. Maitland NJ, Cox MF, Lynas C, Prime SS, Meanwell CA, Scully C. Detection of human papillomavirus DNA in biopsies of human oral tissue. Br J Cancer. 1987 Sep; 56(3):245-50.

41. Bagan JV, Gonzalez L, Milain MA, Lloria E, Cardona F, Jimenez Y. Preliminary investigation of the association of oral lichen planus and hepatitis C. Oral Surg Oral Med Oral Pathol Oral Radiol Endod. 1998; 85:532-6

42. Carrozzo M, Brancatello F, Dametto E, Arduino P, Pentenero M, Rendine S, Porter SR, Lodi G, Scully C, Gandolfo S. Hepatitis C virus-associated oral lichen planus: is the geographical heterogeneity related to HLA-DR6? J Oral Pathol Med. 2005 Apr; 34(4):204-8.

43. Rojo-Moreno JL, Bagán JV, Rojo-Moreno J, Donat JS, Milián MA, Jiménez Y. Psychologic factors and oral lichen planus. A psychometric evaluation of 100 cases. Oral Surg Oral Med Oral Pathol Oral Radiol Endod. 1998 Dec; 86(6):687-91.

44. Rodstrom PO, Ibbotson SH, Speight EL, Macleod RI, Smart ER, Lawrence CM. The relevance and effect of amalgam replacement in subjects with oral lichenoid reactions. Br J Dermatol. 1996 Mar; 134(3):420-3.

45. Ivanovski K, Nakova M, Warburton G, Pesevska S, Filipovska A, Nares S, Nunn ME, Angelova D, Angelov N. Psychological profile in oral lichen planus. J Clin Periodontol. 2005 Oct; 32(10):1034-40.

46. McCartan BE, Lamey PJ. Expression of CD1 and HLA-DR by Langerhans cells (LC) in oral lichenoid drug eruptions (LDE) and idiopathic oral lichen planus (LP). J Oral Pathol Med. 1997 Apr; 26(4):176-80.

47. Femiano F, Scully C. Functions of the cytokines in relation oral lichen planus-hepatitis C. Med Oral Patol Oral Cir Bucal. 2005 Apr 1;10

48. Montebugnoli L, Farnedi A, Marchetti C, Magrini E, Pession A, Foschini MP. High proliferative activity and chromosomal instability in oral lichen planus. Int J Oral Maxillofac Surg. 2006 Dec; 35(12):1140-4.

49. Tao XA, Li CY, Xia J, Yang X, Chen XH, Jian YT, Cheng B. Differential gene expression profiles of whole lesions from patients with oral lichen planus. J Oral Pathol Med. 2009 May; 38(5):427-33.

50. Yarom N, Dagon N, Shinar E, Gorsky M. Association between hepatitis C virus infection and oral lichen planus in Israeli patients. Isr Med Assoc J. 2007 May; 9(5):370-2.

51. Silverman S, Gorsky M, Lozada-Nur F. A prospective follow-up study of 570 patients with oral lichen planus persistence, remission and malignant association. Oral Surg Oral Med Oral Pathol 1985;60:30-4.

52. Gasco M, Crook T. The p53 network in head and neck cancer. *Oral Oncology*. 2003;39(3):222–231.

53. Ebrahimi M, Nylander K, van der Waal I. Oral lichen planus and the p53 family: what do we know? *Journal of Oral Pathology and Medicine*. 2011;40(4):281–285.

54. Meek DW. The p53 response to DNA damage. *DNA Repair*. 2004;3(8-9):1049–1056.

55. Safadi RA, Jaber SZA, Hammad HM, Hamasha AAH. Oral lichen planus shows higher expressions of tumor suppressor gene products of p53 and p21 compared to oral mucositis. An immunohistochemical study. *Archives of Oral Biology*. 2010;55(6):454–461.

56. Chaiyarit P, Ma N, Hiraku Y, et al. Nitrative and oxidative DNA damage in oral lichen planus in relation to human oral carcinogenesis. *Cancer Science*. 2005;96(9):553–559.

57. Lee JJ, Kuo MY, Cheng SJ, et al. Higher expressions of p53 and proliferating cell nuclear antigen (PCNA) in atrophic oral lichen planus and patients with areca quid chewing. *Oral Surgery, Oral Medicine, Oral Pathology, Oral Radiology, and Endodontology*. 2005;99(4):471–478.

58. Bartkova J, Rezaei N, Liontos M, et al. Oncogene-induced senescence is part of the tumorigenesis barrier imposed by DNA damage checkpoints. *Nature*. 2006;444(7119):633–637.

59. Gorgoulis VG, Vassiliou LVF, Karakaidos P, et al. Activation of the DNA damage checkpoint and genomic instability in human precancerous lesions. *Nature*. 2005;434(7035):907–913.

60. Zhang L, Michelsen C, Cheng X, Zeng T, Priddy R, Rosin MP. Molecular analysis of oral lichen planus: a premalignant lesion? *American Journal of Pathology*. 1997;151(2):323–327.

61. Zhang L, Cheng X, Li YH, et al. High frequency of allelic loss in dysplastic lichenoid lesions. *Laboratory Investigation*. 2000;80(2):233–237.

62. Kim J, Yook JI, Lee EH, et al. Evaluation of premalignant potential in oral lichen planus using interphase cytogenetics. *Journal of Oral Pathology and Medicine*. 2001;30(2):65–72.

63. Accurso BT, Warner BM, Knobloch TJ, et al. Allelic imbalance in oral lichen planus and assessment of its classification as a premalignant condition. *Oral Surgery, Oral Medicine, Oral Pathology, Oral Radiology, and Endodontology*. 2011;112(3):359–366.

64. Femiano F, Scully C. DNA cytometry of oral leukoplakia and oral lichen planus. *Medicina Oral Patologia Oral y Cirugia Bucal*. 2005;10(supplement 1):E9–E14.

65. Hosni ES, Yurgel LS, Silva VDD. DNA ploidy in oral lichen planus, determined by image cytometry. *Journal of Oral Pathology and Medicine*. 2010;39(3):206–211.

66. Rode M, Flezar MS, Kogoj-Rode M, et al. Image cytometric evaluation of nuclear texture features and DNA content of the reticular form of oral lichen planus. *Analytical & Quantitative Cytology & Histology*. 2006;28(5):262–268.

67. Montebugnoli L, Farnedi A, Marchetti C, Magrini E, Pession A, Foschini MP. High proliferative activity and chromosomal instability in oral lichen planus. *International Journal of Oral and Maxillofacial Surgery*. 2006;35(12):1140–1144.

68. Thongprasom K, Chaimusig M, Korkij W, Sererat T, Luangjarmekorn L, Rojwattanasirivej S. A randomized controlled trial to compare topical cyclosporin with triamcinolone acetonide for the treatment of oral lichen planus. *J Oral Pathol Med*. 2007;36(3):142–146.

69. Cribier B, Frances C, Chosidow O. Treatment of lichen planus. An evidence-based medicine analysis of efficacy. *Arch Dermatol.* 1998;134(12):1521–1530.

70. Corrocher G, Di Lorenzo G, Martinelli N, et al. Comparative effect of tacrolimus 0.1% ointment and clobetasol 0.05% ointment in patients with oral lichen planus. *J Clin Periodontol.* 2008;35(3):244–249.

71. Carbone M, Arduino PG, Carrozzo M, et al. Topical clobetasol in the treatment of atrophic-erosive oral lichen planus: a randomized controlled trial to compare two preparations with different concentrations. *J Oral Pathol Med.* 2009;38(2):227–233.

72. Voûte AB, Schulten EA, Langendijk PN, Kostense PJ, van der Waal I. Fluocinonide in an adhesive base for treatment of oral lichen planus. A double-blind, placebo-controlled clinical study. *Oral Surg Oral Med Oral Pathol.* 1993;75(2):181–185.

73. Lodi G, Scully C, Carrozzo M, Griffiths M, Sugerman PB, Thongprasom K. Current controversies in oral lichen planus: report of an international consensus meeting. Part 2. Clinical management and malignant transformation. *Oral Surg Oral Med Oral Pathol Oral Radiol Endod.* 2005;100(2):164–178.

74. Radfar L, Wild RC, Suresh L. A comparative treatment study of topical tacrolimus and clobetasol in oral lichen planus. *Oral Surg Oral Med Oral Pathol Oral Radiol Endod.* 2008;105(2):187–193.

75. Volz T, Caroli U, Lüdtke H, et al. Pimecrolimus cream 1% in erosive oral lichen planus—a prospective randomized double-blind vehicle-controlled study [published correction appears in Br J Dermatol. 2008;159(4):994]. *Br J Dermatol.* 2008;159(4):936–941.

76. 23. Choonhakarn C, Busaracome P, Sripanidkulchai B, Sarakarn P. The efficacy of aloe vera gel in the treatment of oral lichen planus: a randomized controlled trial. *Br J Dermatol.* 2008;158(3):573–577.

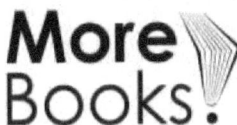
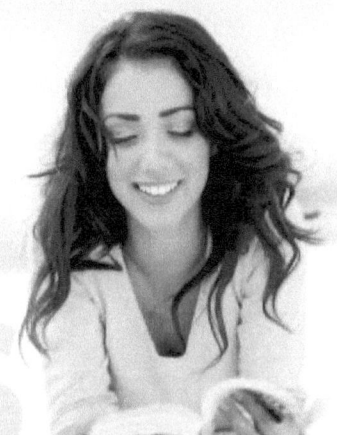

I want morebooks!

Buy your books fast and straightforward online - at one of world's fastest growing online book stores! Environmentally sound due to Print-on-Demand technologies.

Buy your books online at
www.morebooks.shop

Kaufen Sie Ihre Bücher schnell und unkompliziert online – auf einer der am schnellsten wachsenden Buchhandelsplattformen weltweit! Dank Print-On-Demand umwelt- und ressourcenschonend produziert.

Bücher schneller online kaufen
www.morebooks.shop

KS OmniScriptum Publishing
Brivibas gatve 197
LV-1039 Riga, Latvia
Telefax: +371 686 204 55

info@omniscriptum.com
www.omniscriptum.com

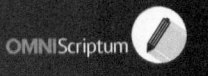

www.ingramcontent.com/pod-product-compliance
Lightning Source LLC
Chambersburg PA
CBHW031538210526
45464CB00003B/1065